The
Flesh Eaters

*The World's Deadliest Flesh-Eating
Diseases*

J.D. Sherwood

Sherwood Publications

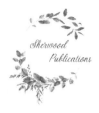

I would like to dedicate this book to my wonderful, inspirational daughter Mahala and loving boyfriend Gabe for encouraging and supporting me throughout this book creation process. And most importantly, my fabulous mom, Fiona, who taught me to believe in myself and to believe that I can do anything I want to in life as long as I try hard enough.

CONTENTS

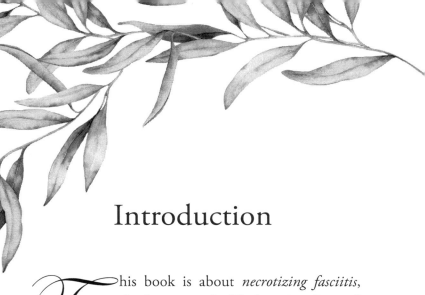

Introduction

This book is about *necrotizing fasciitis*, also known as the "flesh-eating disease." In it, you will find stories of people who have faced death from different forms of the disease and sometimes lost the battle. Let's begin with a few real-life stories that illustrate the horrendous consequences of getting one of these devastating diseases.

It started as a simple toothache, but before his ordeal was over, Peter's life would hang in the balance. At first, when the tooth started bothering him, he ignored it, but eventually, when his face and the floor of his mouth became swollen, Peter decided to go to the dentist. She diagnosed an abscessed tooth and gave Peter a prescription for antibiotics.

Next, Peter's throat closed up, and he struggled to breathe. With his tongue, he could feel a cut behind his tooth. Every ten minutes, it was secreting offensive brown gunk. Peter was forced to spit it into a cup, which soon filled with foul-tasting fluid. It had the odor of decaying flesh. That's because it was dying flesh. Peter's neck and throat were being invaded by necrotizing fasciitis. The doctors put in a breathing tube but couldn't guarantee that Peter would live.

Surgeons tried to remove the dead tissue and encountered handfuls of black goo in his throat. The incision extended from Peter's mouth all the way down to his collarbones. His illness required multiple surgeries in order to remove all the dead and dying flesh. Peter was left with a gaping hole in his throat, exposing his muscles and even his esophagus. For the wound to heal properly, he had to have muscle and skin grafts from his chest. In the end, Peter was left with a grotesque scar that looked as if his throat had been cut.

Kate's left leg was swelling up from her knee down, twice the size of her right leg, so badly that the pressure on her skin was intense. At first, even the doctors paid little attention, not even giving her pain medication. But Kate had an abscess, a collection of pus under the skin, and it kept growing larger and larger. The many medications doctors tried did nothing to slow its progress, and they argued whether this could be a strep or staph infection. Whatever it was, it was definitely antibiotic-resistant, forming another abscess.

Every day, the nurses had to clean the wounds. But

this wasn't a gentle cleansing with a sponge and some antibiotic ointment. It required using a scalpel to cut and scrape away the dead tissue that was spreading throughout her leg, a process that causes excruciating pain. Every day, her flesh was cut away as the infection ravaged Kate's body. Kate was losing more and more muscle tissue as they continued to cut. The doctors discussed amputating her leg. At last, the abscesses burst, and blood and pus drenched Kate's leg. In a way, it was a relief to be free of the awful pressure that had built up as the abscesses grew and Kate's leg swelled.

After two months of terrifying symptoms and painful treatments, Kate finally was able to go home. She had just survived necrotizing fasciitis, a deadly disease that could easily have killed her.

Carolyn, a resident of Florida, had a similar story—but with a much worse outcome. Her ordeal started with a visit to a beach, where she stumbled and got a small cut on her shin. The cut was bandaged, and Carolyn thought no more about it until a few days later, when it became painful. She went to an urgent care facility to have them examine her leg, which by this time was red and swollen. They gave her a tetanus shot and an antibiotic. Neither of them would have any effect.

Friends who came to deliver the prescription found

Carolyn unconscious on the floor; her left shin completely black. She was hospitalized and diagnosed with necrotizing fasciitis, a flesh-eating disease that ravages the human body, causing the death of enormous amounts of tissue and blasting the human immune system as it poisons the blood and leads to septic shock. Carolyn required several surgeries in a desperate attempt to stop the infection's relentless progress. But her entire body became septic, and she suffered two strokes and kidney failure. Two weeks after her minor injury, Carolyn died. Her grieving family shared her story in an attempt to alert others to the deadly dangers of necrotizing fasciitis and prevent another tragedy such as Carolyn's.

Another death shocked the whole world and spread awareness of necrotizing fasciitis. Beloved entertainer Jim Henson, creator of the Muppets, lost a battle with the disease. In his case, the bacteria invaded his lungs, causing necrotizing pneumonia. There is no vaccine against the Group A streptococcus that killed Henson—or any other form of the disease, which can be caused by a wide variety of bacteria.

Flesh-eating diseases plague the world. They appear in every country and every climate; in every age group from infants to seniors; and throughout beaches, lakes, forests, and your own backyard. They're transmitted in any number of ways—person-to-person, animal-to-human, and even from the soil and water that surround us all. They cause untold suffering, disfigurement, and, in many cases, death.

Flesh-eating diseases also fascinate us. While you never want to get one yourself, you can't seem to look away when someone else gets one. Why? Part of it is the sheer terror they produce. Like good horror movies, the feelings you get make you shudder. Like good medical shows, these stories involve you in life-and-death dramas. And like any compelling personal story, they let you experience all the emotions—sadness, courage, and sometimes even triumph.

But what are flesh-eating diseases, really? The name "necrotizing fasciitis" comes from the Greek word "*nekros*," which means relating to a corpse or death; the word "*fascia*," which is a fibrous connective tissue that supports muscles throughout the body; and "*itis*," which means inflammation (Etymology Online). Necrotizing fasciitis is an infection that results in the fascia becoming inflamed, resulting in the death of surrounding tissues.

Necrotizing fasciitis can destroy skin, fat, and the tissue covering the muscle all within the space of a few hours as the infection rapidly progresses. The chances of survival are slim if a victim doesn't receive appropriate medical care in time. And that treatment usually involves surgery to remove the infected tissue and antibiotics to fight the infection. Sometimes even more drastic measures—including amputation of diseased limbs—are required. Decaying skin, dying tissue, and rotting flesh can add up to a medical mystery that changes lives and frequently ends them.

Many different bacteria can cause flesh-eating diseases. Among them are Group *A streptococcus, Staphylococcus aureus, Vibrio vulnificus, Klebsiella pneumoniae, Clostridium perfringens, Aeromonas hydrophila,* and *Leishmania.* All of them wreak havoc on life and limb. Some of the infectious agents are relatives of other terrifying, fatal diseases such as cholera and botulism.

The flesh-eating bacteria most often enter the body through breaks in the skin, such as cuts and insect bites, but they can also enter through the digestive tract when someone prepares or eats contaminated seafood, for example. Symptoms include a high fever and a red, severely painful swelling that feels hot and spreads rapidly. They're nonspecific and easy to downplay. But as the bacteria multiply and keep invading your body, the skin becomes purplish and then goes black and dies from the extensive tissue destruction. Flesh-eating disease is fatal in 24% to 34% of cases, sometimes in less than 24 hours. Complications such as toxic shock increase the mortality rate to 60% (Christiansen, 2021).

No wonder it strikes fear in the hearts of the people whose lives it touches! Just the words "necrotizing fasciitis" can change your life forever or end it without mercy.

Let's take a closer look at flesh-eating diseases— what they are, how they take over the human body, and how they can kill.

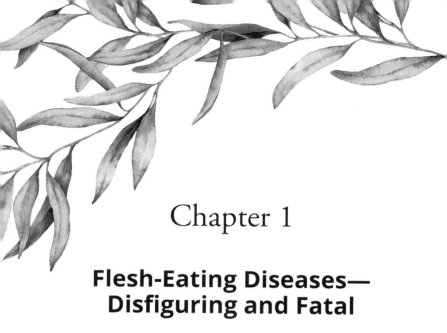

Chapter 1

Flesh-Eating Diseases—
Disfiguring and Fatal

You've heard the stories. You've seen the videos and pictures. You've shuddered at the thought of flesh-eating diseases. The possibility of actually getting one never crossed your mind, although. But the threat is real. Necrotizing fasciitis, the technical term for flesh-eating infections, is more than just something invented for movies and TV. It's a real condition that kills mercilessly and leaves mutilated bodies in its wake.

But what do you really know about necrotizing fasciitis? What are the organisms that cause it? How can you tell if you are infected with it? Can doctors save your life if you get diagnosed with it? Will you be permanently maimed or disfigured? Will you die a hideous death? And can you do anything to lessen the chances that a flesh-eating disease will take over your body, destroy your tissues, and leave you and your family devastated?

We'll be addressing these and other questions as we go through the havoc that flesh-eating diseases cause and the ways they invade and speed through your body.

Real Life Cases

But first, let's look at the deadliest of the organisms and the people who've had to confront their own mortality—and sometimes lose the battle.

Monica came close to death but managed to dodge the bullet of necrotizing fasciitis—though it changed her life forever.

It should have been one of the happiest days of her life. Monica was about to give birth to her second child, a baby girl. The birth seemed to go well at first. But shortly after the C-section she underwent, Monica began to develop a fever. At first, she thought it was nothing to worry about—merely a minor complication of the recent surgical procedure. Next, she felt sharp pains in her abdomen that just kept coming. Before long, Monica was in critical condition and had to be airlifted to another hospital where her illness could be better treated. There she received the life-changing diagnosis of necrotizing fasciitis.

Monica quickly developed septic shock, a drastic condition that happens when a severe infection runs rampant throughout the body, causing blood pressure to fall dramatically. Bodily organs can't get enough oxygen and begin to shut down. By itself, septic shock is life-threatening, but combined with necrotizing fasciitis, it's practically a death sentence.

Trying to get the infection under control, doctors were forced to make some drastic choices. Cutting away the dead and dying tissue, they removed Monica's uterus, ovaries, gallbladder, and most of her colon. She would never be able to have more children—but now the most important consideration became saving her life. Doctors stabilized Monica, but they realized that even more devastating surgery would be necessary.

All four of Monica's limbs needed to be amputated because the infection had killed off their tissue. There was no way to save her arms and legs. More than 35 surgeries were necessary to cut away all the dead tissue and remove all four of her limbs. Without her arms and legs, Monica had to learn to care for her new baby with the help of rehabilitation services.

Len, who lived in the Outer Banks of North Carolina, was out in his yard gardening, as he often did, on Labor Day weekend. He didn't realize that he was about to have a brush with death. Len wasn't wearing gardening gloves and felt a small prick on his thumb. He wasn't overly concerned, but he did clean and bandage the wound.

A day later, Len decided to do some cleaning up and empty the storm drains around his house, which had been damaged in a hurricane. Afterward, he noticed that the seemingly insignificant injury on his thumb had grown red and sensitive. His wife treated the site with antibacterial ointment and a clean dressing. But it was too late. The bacteria were already multiplying in his system. The next day, his thumb was seriously discolored and swollen, and it became progressively worse as the day went on.

That afternoon, Len went to the hospital, where he had a variety of tests and x-rays. Doctors started antibiotic therapy, but it didn't really do anything. Len visited an urgent care clinic the next day. The wound was even more swollen and had begun to turn black. A red line had developed, reaching from his hand to his armpit, an indication that the infection was rapidly spreading throughout his bloodstream. The medical personnel told him to return to the hospital immediately.

The doctor at the hospital did more tests and gave Len more antibiotics. He recognized that the infection was out of control and called in another doctor who had more experience with this kind of illness. She recognized that the infection was potentially devastating, started intravenous antibiotics, and referred Len to an infectious disease specialist and a hand surgeon. He was then sent to the emergency room at the facility where they practiced.

The specialists realized immediately that Len was suffering from necrotizing fasciitis and began treatment right away. Five days later, Len was well enough to be released. His hand was saved, and the infection was at last under control. But six weeks later, he said that he was still not fully recovered. It would take until the end of the year for him to get back to most of his former strength.

The Deadly Culprits

There are a number of different organisms that can cause necrotizing fasciitis and lead to death or disfigurement. You'll learn about many of them in the following chapters, but for now, let's take a look at some of the most common.

Streptococcus A

Streptococcus A is an organism that nearly everyone has experience with. It's the reason that so many people get strep throat from time to time. Strep throat isn't usually deadly, but when it turns into a runaway infection, it can be a life-threatening hazard. In fact, *Streptococcus A* is the most common cause of necrotizing fasciitis. Because it often starts with flu-like symptoms, sometimes it takes a while until it is recognized that a flesh-eating disease has taken hold and is running rampant through the body. And that delay can mean the difference between life and death.

Case Studies

Reign, a four-year-old girl in England, contracted *Streptococcus A* as a complication of chickenpox. She barely survived.

A few days after Reign contracted chickenpox, her mother noticed that her daughter was suffering from a fever and extreme exhaustion. Then she noticed that there was a red ring developing around one of Reign's chickenpox sores. She took Reign to the emergency room to get antibiotics. But the red ring had continued to grow, tripling in size. The doctors did supply antibiotics but told the mother to take her daughter home;

with the excuse that they were too busy, and Reign was too infectious.

Reign's mother took her to another hospital, where she had to wait six hours to be seen, despite the fact that the little girl's condition was going rapidly downhill. She was nearly lifeless; her temperature had gone up to a dangerous 107°F, and she was hallucinating from the fever.

Finally, after she was diagnosed with necrotizing fasciitis caused by *Streptococcus A*, Reign was rushed into the operating room. The surgeons made a large incision in her side to remove the deteriorating flesh and prevent the infection from spreading even further. But Reign was not responding after the surgery, so she was sent to the ICU, where she was put into a medically induced coma and started on a breathing machine. The doctors explained that the infection had raged throughout her body and had caused her whole system to teem with bacteria. It was not certain that she could survive.

After three weeks in the hospital, Reign miraculously recovered, and her mother took her home. But the little girl had a terrible souvenir—a huge scar where the doctors had operated on her. Reign's mother has shared her horrific story publicly to let others know how quickly a seemingly common illness could become a life-threatening condition. It wasn't the chickenpox that almost killed her daughter—it was *Streptococcus A* bacteria and necrotizing fasciitis.

In Lebanon, a 19-year-old boy fell off a skateboard, suffering several scrapes that turned into an inflamed wound with blisters within 24 hours after his accident. A few days later, he went to the hospital. Doctors examined him and found that his lower left leg was extremely swollen and showed signs of dying skin. Soon, it became apparent that the infection was traveling rapidly throughout his body and that he was suffering from necrotizing fasciitis. Tissue cultures showed strep. Powerful antibiotics were given, and the young man was transferred to the ICU.

A day after he was admitted, surgeons cleaned out the man's wound surgically in multiple two-hour sessions, removing muscle tissue that was dead or dying and leaving bloody but living areas of flesh. Still, there were pockets of infection that the doctors couldn't reach, and his leg had to be opened up all the way to his hip for further surgery. His leg looked like one gigantic raw piece of steak. Stronger antibiotics were prescribed, and two weeks later, he was transferred to another hospital.

The young man then underwent extensive skin grafts to try to close the long, deep wound from his ankle to high on his thigh. Doctors who wrote up the case noted that if surgery to clean the wound of dying tissue is delayed for even a couple of hours, the patient is much less likely to survive. They also said that, frequently, a patient with necrotizing fasciitis first enters the hospital through the internal medicine department rather than immediately into surgery because the infection has already started traveling throughout the body. This makes a delay in the treatment more likely.

Vibrio Vulnificus

Although not as common as *Streptococcus A*, *Vibrio vulnificus* is another cause of necrotizing fasciitis that often appears in warm saltwater near beaches and in the southern US. It releases an enzyme that causes flesh to rot away.

Case Studies

A man from Memphis was vacationing in Florida. He died from flesh-eating bacteria 48 hours after swimming in Florida's bays. A 12-year-old girl had died from necrotizing fasciitis after swimming in the same area, but the news reported that she had had a cut on her leg. The man thought that because he didn't have an obvious open wound, he was safe. But he had forgotten about some small scratches on his arms and legs. He thought that they were completely healed.

Twelve hours after enjoying his time at the beach, the man woke up with chills, a fever, and cramping in the abdomen. The family decided to take him home, where he could consult with his regular doctors. On the way, he became dramatically worse, and when he got to the hospital in Memphis, the man had a reddened, swollen sore. His daughter informed the medical personnel that he had been swimming in an area where a girl had gotten sick and died from necrotizing fasciitis. They replied that the media reports were overblown and that the man simply had a staph infection.

The woman's father was transferred to the ICU when his condition continued to deteriorate, but it was too late. When his test results came back—after his death—they showed that he had died from the flesh-eating bacteria *Vibrio vulnificus*, one of the many organisms that can cause the flesh-eating disease.

The daughter, bereft at the loss of her father, publicized the story to warn other people of the dangers. She began campaigning for bacteria alerts to be posted at beaches.

Kenny was a 53-year-old Delaware man who was allergic to seafood but loved cooking crabs for friends. Then one day, he felt a crab fighting back, pinching his hand. He poured rubbing alcohol on it. A co-worker checked on Kenny the next morning, worried that he might be having an allergic reaction to the shellfish. But what was really happening was that the barely visible wound meant that Kenny was infected with *Vibrio vulnificus.*

Two days after the crab pinched Kenny, he had a blood blister on his hand as big as a tangerine, was feverish, and generally felt unwell. He struggled to get dressed and almost fell over when he bent over to tie his shoes. The longer he waited to get help, the worse it got. Soon purple lines were spreading past his wrist, and he became too weak to walk. His body started to swell, too, and he lapsed into unconsciousness. When he got to the hospital, he fell into a coma. He had all the telltale signs of a flesh-eating disease. The doctors recognized the danger and started Kenny on antibiotics—though there aren't many that work on the Vibrio *vulnificus* bacteria.

Four days later, Kenny woke up in intensive care. He found his bandaged hand looking as large as a baseball mitt. He had been on life support for two days and had almost certainly experienced fatal shock; his blood pressure was also very low. But although he had regained consciousness, Kenny was not out of the woods yet. The bacteria were still eating away at his hand. Doctors thought that, even though he pulled through the shock, his hand would never be useful again. Amputation seemed like the only possibility.

Kenny had two surgeries in an attempt to stop the bacteria in its tracks. After he was transferred to another hospital, he had three more. His nerves and other tissues seemed beyond repair. When the bandages finally came off, he was looking at a gaping wound that showed tendons and ligaments. His flesh had been removed to the bone.

When Kenny was finally able to start rehab, he found that the disease had affected his whole arm, right up to the shoulder. His slow progress took place over nine months. And his doctors told him that he had done exactly the wrong thing all those months ago when he poured alcohol on the wound. It would have been better, it seems, if he had instead squeezed it to push the blood and some of the bacteria out.

Klebsiella Pneumoniae

Klebsiella pneumoniae is more often the cause of pneumonia, as the name implies, but it can, under certain circumstances, lead to necrotizing fasciitis. A Seattle hospital recently reported an increase in *Klebsiella pneumoniae* infections, including cases involving wounds and surgical incisions. A variety called "hyper-mucoviscous" *Klebsiella* is particularly dangerous, especially when combined with another bacteria like strep. *Klebsiella pneumoniae* is something we all have within us—it is part of the normal bacteria present in the human gut. But when it spreads out of control, *Klebsiella pneumoniae* can become a flesh-eating nightmare.

Case Studies

While necrotizing fasciitis most often attacks the arms and legs or abdomen, *Klebsiella pneumoniae* can also eat away the flesh of the head or neck, as one 48-year-old Chinese man found out. He thought he was only suffering from a sore throat and fever, but when it lasted four days, he sought treatment at an Ear, Nose, and Throat (ENT) department. When doctors examined him, he had swelling on the left side of his neck, one tonsil, and the roof of his mouth, and he couldn't open his mouth very far. The medical personnel tried to get pus from the swellings but couldn't.

The next day, the man's condition worsened. The swellings were making it difficult for him to breathe. He needed a tracheotomy—a breathing tube placed into his neck—and doctors made an incision under the jaw to drain the area. This time, they found some foul-smelling, grayish-brown pus. Drainage tubes and feeding tubes were put in place, and the patient was transferred to the ICU.

After the surgeries, the patient's face was still extremely swollen, and he was running a fever. The bottom of the man's tongue was not only swollen but ulcerated and oozing pus. It was obvious he had a deep abscess. Samples of the pus were taken, and they showed klebsiella and strep infections.

It wasn't until nine days after the man entered the hospital that his fever broke. It took five more days until the production of pus decreased and he was able to open his mouth normally. Another surgery to clean the wound of dead tissue was needed before the incision could be stitched shut. He finally left the hospital after 37 days of fighting the *Klebsiella pneumoniae* infection.

After three days of suffering with a swollen neck, a 56-year-old man in Japan went to the ER. The warm, tender swelling kept getting worse over the next few days, extending down to his collarbone, and the man couldn't swallow food easily. Within a matter of hours, his blood pressure dropped sharply, and he was taken to the operating room to have a breathing tube inserted in his horribly swollen neck.

Doctors suspected that the man was in septic shock

and possibly had an abscess in his neck, so they rushed him to the ICU. They gave him medications to support his blood pressure. The swelling that had reached his collarbone by now had reached his shoulder and chest, with mottled purple and blue skin and blisters. At that point, doctors considered the diagnosis of necrotizing fasciitis. Surgeons were consulted who might be able to operate on the man to remove dead tissue and drain the abscess, but the surgery would have been too close to the man's spine to be safe.

It was too late for the Japanese man, however. Only 24 hours after he came to the ER, he died of cardiac arrest brought on by his illness. Testing revealed that the man had been suffering from the most vicious form of *Klebsiella pneumoniae*—but by that time, it was much too late.

Clostridium Perfringens

Clostridium perfringens is a sneaky organism. It can change from needing oxygen in order to grow to surviving without oxygen. This makes it adaptable to many different environments. It hides in the human body, living harmlessly in the gut or urinary tract until it grows at several inches per hour and colonizes other areas, destroying tissue as it goes.

Gas gangrene—another name for necrotizing

fasciitis—results when bodily tissues are riddled with gas that the bacteria produce. The toxins that *Clostridium perfringens* produces damage the tissues— that's what produces the gas. Large black bubbles of gas appear along with the purpling and blackening of the skin.

It's not always possible to tell how *Clostridium perfringens* enters the body. Often, there isn't a puncture or scratch. But the infection moves rapidly and can lead to multiorgan failure. Doctors can mistake gastric gangrene for cellulitis at first, making diagnosis difficult. X-rays and CTs don't reveal the pockets of gas until it's too late.

Discharge from the area that looks like dishwater or fat that peels easily away from the tissue is something that doctors should be on the lookout for. The only treatment is to cut away the dead tissue. The surgeon will know that the dead flesh is gone when they reach live, bleeding, red tissue. Then, reconstructive surgery, such as skin grafts, will be required to cover the places where dead tissue was cut away. It's a process that often takes months. And that's if the patient survives.

A 17-year-old girl, who was previously quite healthy, came to a local clinic when she fell off her chair at school. She got a small scratch and a sharp pain somewhere in her left hand. The doctors suspected a broken bone, so they put her hand and lower arm in a cast. It was the wrong thing to do.

One week later, the cast hadn't helped, and an x-ray showed no broken bones. By this time, the young woman was in intolerable pain. When the cast was removed, doctors found the back of her hand was swollen and included an even larger raised central area that looked like a puckered scar. Around it, the skin was mottled purple. A few days after the cast was removed, the swelling was so severe that you couldn't even see her knuckles. The skin still looked mottled. It was clear that gas was accumulating on the back of her hand.

After a transfer to another hospital, a piece of the woman's skin was harvested and taken away for a biopsy. It revealed the bacteria Clostridium perfringens. She was given antibiotics for a total of 22 days with no improvement. In fact, the disease had progressed to involve her face, right hand, trunk, left leg, and shoulder blade. It was time for more drastic action. Doctors wanted to amputate her hand, but her parents refused. Five surgeries were attempted to cut away the dead flesh, and more antibiotics were given, to no avail.

Hyperbaric oxygen therapy, which involves lying in a special chamber while 100% oxygen is pumped in, began. This lets the lungs send more oxygen to the body parts that need it. Getting more oxygen to the tissues helps them heal. It helped her condition for a while, but after 40 treatments, the woman experienced intolerable side effects, including ear blockage, pain in her neck and arms, and bleeding from her scalp. After 139 treatments plus antibiotics, her condition hadn't improved. If nothing changed, her chances of dying were high.

Another Clostridium patient was a 56-year-old woman from Texas who came to the emergency room after suffering for two days from pain, discoloration, and swelling in her right hand. It might have been an infection in her blood, the doctors thought, so they gave her antibiotics and IV fluids. She was transferred to the ICU for further treatment.

They gave the woman a CT scan, which suggested that her disease was a flesh-eating one that extended into her forearm as well as her hand. The skin on her fingers was tight and plump as sausages, and black and purple mottling marred her hand, indicating that the tissue there was dying. Six days later, her lower leg, foot, and toes were involved too, with black, gas-filled blisters.

The woman went into septic shock when the bacteria poisoned her bloodstream and flooded throughout her body. Doctors rushed her to the operating room and performed an emergency amputation of her arm just below the elbow. They continued treating her with penicillin and other antibiotics, but the infection just continued to spread into her vital organs. Her heart, lungs, digestive system, and kidney system were all beginning to fail. At last, the bloodwork came back with a diagnosis of *Clostridium perfringens* rather than the MRSA the doctors had suspected.

Because of the woman's multiorgan failure and her worsening condition, a decision was made to simply make her comfortable, and she died after eight days of suffering from gas gangrene.

E. coli

The *E. coli* bacteria has become notorious for causing serious and even deadly illnesses when someone eats raw vegetables or undercooked meat or drinks contaminated water. The bacteria usually result in gastrointestinal illness with abdominal pain and diarrhea, but sometimes the toxins produced by the bacteria cause life-threatening kidney failure. And sometimes, *E. coli* causes necrotizing fasciitis.

A 29-year-old woman was referred to an intensive care unit suffering, everyone believed, from septic shock from bacteria that had been transported throughout her body by her infected blood. For four days previously, she had a fever and pain in her left leg. Doctors had treated her with steroids.

Next, the woman developed a purple-mottled area on the back of her left thigh, extending down below her knee. Broad-spectrum antibiotics were started, but CT scans of her leg and abdomen revealed involvement in the tissue beneath her skin. It was becoming obvious that she was suffering from necrotizing fasciitis. Doctors had to cut away the dead flesh until they reached areas of tissue that were still alive.

The samples of blood and tissue from the surgery showed the presence of E. coli bacteria, and different antibiotics were tried, to no avail. The woman went into kidney failure, and the surgical wound continued bleeding, necessitating huge transfusions, but her condition only worsened. A day later, the surgery had to be repeated. Soft tissue death had now reached the woman's whole thigh. Blood flowed like a river as the surgeons tried their best to clear away the dying tissue. They were unsuccessful and the woman died during the second surgery.

Staphylococcus Aureus

Staphylococcus aureus infections usually affect the skin.

Some infections go away on their own, while others need to be treated with antibiotics. They can also cause more serious problems like blood poisoning, toxic shock syndrome, and necrotizing fasciitis.

It didn't start out looking too alarming. The 61-year-old man waited two months before he reported redness and swelling in his legs. He thought it might be a flare-up of his gout, a painful form of inflammatory arthritis. The drugs he was given for gout had caused a rash all across his body, along with scratches, ulceration, and scabs. The man was given anti-allergy drugs. When the rash disappeared, he was sent home.

However, an ultrasound and MRI of his legs showed swelling of the soft tissue and a possible abscess in the muscle. Bloody, pus-filled fluid was drained from the abscess. Examining the pus and blood confirmed that an infection with *Staphylococcus aureus* was the cause. Every day, pus flowed from the drainage tube. Another MRI found that the swelling and abscesses were getting worse. Within two days, the man needed to have the dying tissue cut away. The flesh appeared gray, and pus-filled fluid was still present. A week later, the process was repeated. Still, his right leg failed to heal.

Before a third surgery could be done, the man coughed up bloody fluid, and his lungs started wheezing. The infection had made it to his lungs. Then, it reached his heart. Aggressive treatment was tried, and it did help, but more surgery on his infected leg was delayed while the infection continued to spread. Eventually, he had six more sessions of cutting away the dead tissue, once a week. Skin grafts were needed to close the wounds. After four months in the hospital, the man was released.

Aeromonas Hydrophila

Yet another organism that can cause flesh-eating disease is *Aeromonas hydrophila*. It destroys healthy tissue, even when doctors act aggressively to slow or stop the spread, and can lead to death.

Aimee, 24 years old, was vacationing at the Little Tallapoosa River, near Atlanta. She was riding a jury-rigged zipline when it broke, and she fell. The severe injury to her calf that she suffered required 22 staples to close.

Three days later, Aimee was still feeling pain, so she went to a local emergency room. The doctors took little time to realize that she was suffering from necrotizing fasciitis. They discovered that the cause was the bacteria

Aeromonas hydrophila. Their quick action probably saved her life.

It couldn't save her from further trauma, though. The young woman went into multi-organ failure and needed a respirator to breathe for her. Her kidneys failed, and she went on full-time dialysis. Her heart was barely beating.

Surgeons tried to remove dead tissue at the site where the bacteria entered the body, all the way down to healthy tissue, but it was no use. Despite their efforts to prevent the bacteria from moving through Aimee's body, they were unsuccessful. The surgeons had to amputate most of her hands. They also cut away part of her abdomen, one leg at the hip, and the other foot.

Aimee has made the best of her situation by becoming an advocate for people with disabilities. Recently, she posted to social media a picture of herself in a bathing suit, with her missing limbs, scars, and skin grafts proudly on display.

Chapter 2

The Most Feared Skin Disease

*J*ust the word leprosy strikes fear in the hearts of people around the world. The disease's fearsome reputation goes back to biblical times and even further. For thousands of years, it was both disfiguring and incurable, believed to be the result of a curse, heredity, or even a punishment for sin. People with awful skin lesions and missing body parts were considered unclean and shunned by the uninfected. Sufferers were quarantined or driven away from inhabited areas, left to themselves to live or die. Leprosy has also been called the "scourge of humanity."

The Devastation of Leprosy

Leprosy ravaged Europe and the Middle East throughout the Dark Ages. There's no telling how many people have died from the disease, but every year there are still more than 200,000 cases in 120 countries around the world, despite the World Health Organization's attempts to eradicate leprosy (2023). Areas with overcrowding, malnutrition, and poor sanitation have always been—and still are—places where leprosy thrives. Leprosy reached the Americas as a result of the slave trade.

Leprosy is now also called Hansen's Disease, after the doctor who finally saw the leprosy bacteria under a microscope about 150 years ago. The bacteria infects the skin, leading to disfiguring lesions and damaging the nerves. It grows best in cooler places, so the places away from the central core of the body—ears, nose, fingers, and toes—are the most likely sites for the disease to flourish. Discolored, insensitive patches of skin on the face and body are an early symptom. Many diseases can cause skin discoloration, but only leprosy leaves the flesh insensitive to the touch.

The affected parts lose their blood supply, blacken, rot, and are reabsorbed into the body. In the early days, it was incurable, which explains the horror and disgust with which people viewed lepers. Extremely painful injections of Chaulmoogra oil were the only treatment that held out any hope, but they were largely unsuccessful.

Nerve damage to the hands and feet means that they become insensitive to pain, allowing the extremities to be damaged when the person doesn't realize that they've been injured. These unnoticed injuries lead to other infections and ulcers that progress to gangrene and add to the disfigurement and loss of body parts. Even the eyes can be damaged if they are scratched, leading to blindness. Muscle weakness and paralysis are also possible. The hands can curl into claw-like positions, and the eyes may not be able to close.

Someone can be infected with leprosy and not realize it for years. The bacteria lie in wait inside the body, gradually causing damage. A person who is infected can spread the disease by sneezing or coughing. Although for a long time it was thought that leprosy could be transmitted with a simple touch, it really requires being in close contact with an infected person over a long period of time.

Leprosy Still Exists

Cody, a 14-year-old Texas boy, began to feel weak instead of his usual energetic self. And his body was covered by a red rash. His mother thought he probably had measles, but the doctors she took him to noted that he didn't have the fever that accompanies the infection. Measles was thought to have been eliminated from the US in 2000, but outbreaks can occur because some children don't receive vaccinations, especially now that it seems to have been eradicated. Still, measles wasn't the problem that afflicted Cody.

Cody was embarrassed by the rash that covered his body and by his weakness and lethargy. Kids at school wondered what was wrong with him and so did his family. After two years of visiting doctor after doctor, Cody was no better. In fact, he suddenly became worse. His brother noticed one morning that Cody's spots had ulcerated and broken open. They oozed blood and pus from the blackish holes. They were painful and getting worse.

At the hospital, the doctors feared that Cody had contracted a flesh-eating disease. They ran multiple tests and found that his blood, liver, and kidney counts were way down. After all, the skin serves as a barrier to infection, and when it's compromised, various organisms can enter the body and cause disease.

But Cody's lesions weren't caused by an infection that entered his body. Rather, the oozing lesions were a symptom that an infection was already ravaging his system. And, when the doctors cut into one of the sores and biopsied it, they were shocked to find that what had caused Cody's illness was a disease that seemed like something from the past—leprosy. It was a shock, but it explained his symptoms. The leprosy bacteria had invaded the muscles beneath the skin, weakening them and explaining his general lack of energy. Cody was lucky that he showed symptoms so soon and that the doctors figured out what was causing them. Diagnosing Cody's illness took only a few years, but leprosy can lie dormant for as much as 20 years before symptoms occur.

Although leprosy responds to modern antibiotics, Cody had experienced symptoms for so long that his body was severely compromised. His lesions would be difficult to eradicate. Emergency surgery to cut them out was the only way to proceed. Even with the surgery, the doctors feared that Cody might never recover. But the surgery proved to be the turning point. With the dying tissue removed, Cody's body was able to fight off the infection.

Leprosy in the US these days is usually due to contact between people and infected animals—armadillos, to be specific. Cody and his brother had been out in the woods with their dog when it killed an armadillo. That was most likely when Cody came into contact with the creature's blood and contracted the seemingly unlikely disease.

Cody survived his bout with leprosy, but he didn't escape unscathed. He was left with long, deep scars from the surgery and dark, discolored patches on his face and legs where the infection had spread. But at least he was alive.

Leprosy in the US

Leprosy has a long history throughout the world. Even now, most cases of leprosy occur in countries other than those in North America. But people in the US are not immune to the "scourge of humanity." In fact, there's quite a history of leprosy here.

A Hero Among Lepers

Who would voluntarily put themselves at risk of contracting leprosy? Strange as it may seem, there is one man who did just that—and came down with the dreaded disease. But along the way, Father Damien proved a compassionate friend, spiritual guide, and tireless advocate for the inhabitants of the Hawaiian leper colony in the late 1800s. Eventually, he gave his life while serving the people he cared for. He has been an inspiration to many people, including author Robert Louis Stevenson and Mahatma Gandhi, and has been canonized by the Catholic Church as the patron saint of people with leprosy and HIV.

Father Damien was born Jozef de Veuster in Belgium. He joined a monastery, and when Hawaii pleaded for someone to come and help them in their good works, Father Damien heeded the call and traveled there. After a number of years as a missionary, he decided to dedicate the rest of his life to helping the sick.

Hawaiian lepers were living segregated from the rest of the population in a "settlement colony" on the Hawaiian island of Molokai. They received basic supplies such as food and clothing from the Board of Health, but no actual health care. Relatives could visit if they dared, but had to interact with their family members through a chicken wire screen.

Various plans were suggested in which priests would spend two weeks at a time at the colony because they feared the disease, but in 1864, Father Damien volunteered to live there full time, knowing that the post would likely be a death sentence.

In addition to providing medical care, Father Damien helped build homes and churches, as well as coffins, bring water to the lepers' homes, and dig graves. He lived with them, ate from the same plates, and addressed his charges as "we lepers." He also advocated for treating his charges with dignity and respect despite their diseases.

In 1884, Father Damien contracted leprosy himself, realizing it when he discovered that the nerves in his feet could no longer detect heat. He would remain on Molokai with the lepers until his death from leprosy in 1889. He was buried in the graveyard behind a small church that he had built for the lepers.

Molokai was home to more than 8,000 lepers over the 150 years or so since it was founded. By 2020, only a handful of sufferers, many as old as 90, would still live on Molokai.

Where Leprosy in the US Comes From

Although leprosy can be contracted through close personal contact with people who already have the disease, most people in the US do not catch it this way. The people who do come down with leprosy, like Cody, get it from armadillos.

Armadillos are a reservoir—a "disease vector"—of leprosy. They're the only other animal besides humans that can contract the disease in the wild. That's because of the armadillos' naturally low body temperature. In humans, leprosy begins by afflicting the body parts with the lowest temperatures—the extremities such as fingers and toes—that often become disfigured or destroyed by the bacteria.

Nine-banded armadillos live in the Gulf Coast states of the US, like Texas, Louisiana, and Florida. Florida, for example, experiences some cases of leprosy every year. Armadillos can often be seen along the highways. Many times, they are found dead there, as cars run over the small animals. As Cody learned, getting blood from a dead armadillo on you is a real hazard.

One study confirmed that armadillos were "highly likely" to be carriers of the disease and have transmitted it to people (Bruce et al., 2000). People with leprosy were surveyed in a hospital in Houston, and more than 70% of the 69 patients reported contact with armadillos. Another 32 sufferers said they had not had exposure to armadillos, but they were from countries where leprosy is more common and may have caught it through person-to-person contact.

The US Leper Colony That Brought Hope

In Louisiana, where armadillos flourish, there was one leper colony—and research facility—where leprosy was studied and thousands of those with the disease lived. Founded in 1917, the Louisiana Leper Home at Carville provided a place where people with leprosy could live out their lives without confronting the massive stigma that still exists when a person is diagnosed. Fear and loathing from the people of New Orleans led to the creation of Carville.

Many of the people housed there suffered from neuropathy—the nerve damage that the disease causes, leading to the loss of extremities and limbs and disfigurement of the face. With the nerves deadened, the lepers were insensible to injuries that took their body parts. At first, lepers were forced to live in isolation, just as they had been on Molokai. Occasionally, inhabitants would sneak under the fence to escape or to enjoy a brief taste of freedom.

After a cure was found for leprosy, people who lived at Carville were allowed to leave the facility and live elsewhere, but some chose to remain. For many, it had become their home. Now the facility has become a museum and clinical center where Hansen's disease is commemorated and studied. The armadillo was the leprosarium's unofficial mascot. The museum is open to visitors.

Chapter 3

Zombie Fungus—Could It Happen Here?

*Z*ombies are trendy. There are books like *Feed*, movies like *Night of the Comet*, and TV shows like *The Walking Dead* that speculate on what might happen if brain-eating creatures were unleashed on society. Infected and uninfected people would be pitted against each other in a brutal life-or-death struggle. But those are all fictional, right?

Real-Life Zombie Fungi

Millions were horrified when they saw the TV show *The Last of Us*. The plot revolves around a fungus that takes over human beings and converts them into zombie-like creatures. The fungus invades people's brains, and mushroom-like growths and spiky tendrils erupt from their bodies. Society collapses around them in a global pandemic that makes COVID-19 look mild by comparison. With no vaccine and no cure, experts recommend bombing whole cities. In the post-apocalyptic landscape, people turn into savage killers.

The series and the video game it was based on were fictional. But could such a blood-curdling scenario really happen? So far, it hasn't, but someday it might. The writers' and producers' inspiration for their zombie fungus was a real organism that preys on ants.

The zombie ant fungus is called *Ophiocordyceps*. It hijacks the ants' brains and forces them to climb trees and hang there while the fungus eats the ants from the inside out. When the ants die, they release fungal spores that float through the air, eventually landing on other ants and creating more zombie creatures. More than 30 other fungi are also capable of controlling insect brains, including those of butterflies, beetles, and moths, as a way to ensure the perpetuation of their own species.

Are Humans at Risk?

Fortunately, so far, neither *Ophiocordyceps* nor any similar fungus has proven capable of attacking and zombie-fying human beings. But scientists say it's not totally out of the question. They speculate on scenarios in which this could happen.

In particular, people with weakened immune systems—which can happen as a result of HIV infection, chemotherapy, and other conditions—will be particularly vulnerable to invasion by harmful fungi. The continuing rise in new health threats may also make humans more likely to be attacked by a new organism with who-knows-what effects. The COVID-19 pandemic and other recent diseases such as SARS and MERS provide a warning about ignoring the possibility of attack by a new pathogen.

Global warming could be involved in infections as well. As fungi adjust to warmer climates, they become more likely to infect humans because their body temperatures will rise closer to the body heat of people. Once they do infect people, they'll be hard to control because treatments that target the fungi can also be harmful to humans.

Scientists have been rediscovering disease-causing organisms from beneath the permafrost in the Northern Hemisphere, particularly in the Arctic, Siberia, Canada, and Alaska. Permafrost is a layer of soil that occurs in a climate that remains frozen throughout the year. It's also a good place for organisms to survive because it's an environment that is oxygen-free, just like the deep tissues in our bodies. Extinct animals such as mummified mastodons have been recovered from the permafrost, as have at least seven families of viruses. Some of these viruses have been made infectious again.

Not all of these viruses attack humans, but some do. The virus that caused the deadly 1918 flu epidemic that infected 500 million people and killed at least 50 million worldwide. Recent searches for frozen bodies that died during the epidemic have been controversial because of the possibility of reviving the infection and the fact that since that time, people have lost their immunity to it. Anthrax and smallpox have also been isolated from bodies found in the permafrost.

But it isn't just science that threatens to unleash dormant diseases from the permafrost. Climate change keeps accelerating, and the possibility of formerly frozen infectious agents infecting modern populations keeps growing. Computer models indicate that viruses could enter the environment from lakes formed by meltwater from glaciers that have thawed. The danger from these organisms is unknown at the moment, but the consequences could be devastating.

Another Way to Hijack a Brain

Mice cower at the sight of cats. That's the common wisdom. The idea that mice fear cats is supported by thousands of years of observation and is present in all forms of media. Just think about how many cartoons involve mice fleeing from predatory cats. Cats and mice are simply natural enemies.

But there's a brain parasite that can short-circuit that ordinary state of affairs. *Toxoplasma gondii* lives and reproduces in the guts of felines and can infect other animals, including humans. When mice become infected with it, though, their behavior changes. No longer are they afraid of cats. Instead, they don't run away from them as they used to. They lose their fear, which actually makes them more likely to be killed and eaten by cats. The parasite hijacks the mouse's brains for the benefit of the cat.

Once an infected mouse is eaten, the life cycle of the parasite continues, with the cat passing on *T. gondii* in its waste to infect other animals in turn. That's the reason that pregnant women are advised not to clean a cat's litter box—they could easily acquire the parasite, which can cause miscarriage or a stillborn baby. The baby could also suffer brain, liver, or spleen damage or an infection in their eyes. But what if this organism adapted to affect human brains?

Some scientists believe that the effects aren't limited to housecats. They speculate that the parasite makes mice more adventurous and less fearful in general, making them more vulnerable to any species that views them as a tasty snack. Researchers have observed that infected mice also show a lack of fear when exposed to foxes, bobcats, and rats—all of which are extremely predatory when it comes to mice. The mice seem to want to explore more, even in settings that previously would have made them feel threatened.

More Attacks on the Human Brain

While the zombie ant fungus isn't likely to infect the human brain—at least not anytime soon—that doesn't mean there aren't other threats. Any number of other diseases and parasites lurk in the environment, ready to attack.

Naegleria Fowleri

One summer, seven-year-old Kyle was on summer vacation in Texas, happily splashing and swimming in warm river water. What he and his family didn't realize was that, while he was playing, a brain-eating amoeba had gone up his nose and begun to attack the boy's brain.

Three days later, Kyle was playing baseball with his team, unaware that anything was wrong. The very next day, the boy was hit with a fever and a severe headache. He was vomiting too. There was no real cause for alarm, his family thought—it was probably just an ordinary illness such as the stomach flu. But really, the parasite *Naegleria fowleri* had found a way into Kyle's brain through his sinuses.

Soon, however, his parents noticed that Kyle was less responsive and had a dazed look, so they decided to take him to the ER in the local children's hospital. After doctors examined him, they put Kyle into seclusion, fearing that he had bacterial meningitis, a disease that produces inflammation around the outer layers of the brain, causes swelling, and puts pressure on the brain. It's serious—sometimes even fatal—but that wasn't what was happening to Kyle.

The doctors performed a spinal tap on Kyle, inserting a needle into the spinal column and drawing out some of his cerebrospinal fluid. It's an extremely painful procedure. What they found in the fluid was the parasite.

Naegleria fowleri was devouring its way through the lower reaches of Kyle's brain in a route to the brain stem, the part of the brain that controls essential functions like breathing and heart rate. The amoeba was using the brain matter that it ate as fuel to continue its journey closer and closer to the brain stem. When it began eating the tissue of the brain stem, there was no hope. In less than a week after returning from vacation, Kyle died. The parasite *Naegleria fowleri* leads to death in more than 99% of cases (Solis & Cokely, 2010). It's so lethal because it moves rapidly through the brain, doing damage as it eats brain tissue.

A 12-year-old girl named Kali was one of the lucky ones. The amoeba entered her body while she was innocently playing at an Arkansas water park.

The doctors took extreme measures to save her life. They treated her with three different medications that attack fungi and bacteria and an experimental treatment that targets amoebas. They lowered her body temperature to try to slow the rapid progress of the parasite and save her brain tissue. In critical condition, Kali had to have a breathing tube inserted. Eventually, *Naegleria fowleri* was no longer present in her spinal fluid, indicating that the infection had been stopped. After almost 7 weeks since she entered the hospital, including 22 days in the ICU, Kali was finally able to leave.

Her desperate fight for life was successful, but the youngster was left with lingering, significant difficulties. She was able to take only a few steps on her own and had to go through physical and speech therapy, even when she was well enough to return to school.

Naegleria fowleri is found in warm, freshwater locations such as lakes, ditches, hot springs, and swimming pools that aren't properly cared for and chlorinated. Thankfully, it can't be contracted by inadvertently swallowing contaminated water; it must enter the body through the nose and sinuses. Most often, the infection is associated with recreational activities such as swimming and waterskiing. It's most commonly—though not exclusively—found in the southern and southeast parts of the United States, typically during the summer months. The Centers for Disease Control and Prevention (CDC) say to assume that any warm, fresh water contains the amoeba and to take precautions such as keeping your head above water or wearing nose plugs.

Balamuthia Mandrillaris

Balamuthia mandrillaris is another similar infection that invades the brain through the sinuses and produces a disease called Granulomatous Amoebic Encephalitis (GAE). The symptoms can vary from the relatively common fever, headache, and nausea or vomiting, or they can progress to seizures, confusion, and even partial paralysis over weeks to months. GAE is 90% fatal (Amebic Meningitis/Encephalitis, n.d.).

Case Studies

A 26-year-old Hispanic landscape gardener was one of the lucky 10%. He suffered from headaches, visual disturbances, and seizures for two months before he sought treatment. When he did, a brain scan revealed lesions in his brain. Then, when doctors drilled into his skull to take some brain matter for biopsy, the lesions were found to be caused by *Balamuthia mandrillaris*. He most likely got the infection from a skin wound that was infiltrated by the organism, which can live in the soil as well as in water.

For months, he received antimicrobial drugs, but he was not improving, so he was ready to receive "comfort care" in preparation for death. Finally, his brain scans began to clear, and a new antibacterial drug had a positive effect after eight more weeks of therapy. Despite having some toxic effects from the antibiotics, he was completely recovered after two years.

A 69-year-old woman who had a history of chronic sinus infections tried to alleviate her symptoms by using a saline irrigation device. Unfortunately, she didn't follow the recommendations to use distilled water in it. Instead, she used tap water and contracted *Balamuthia mandrillaris*. This wasn't discovered for a long time.

Her early symptom of a scabbed, red sore on her nose were thought to be a skin condition, and the seizures that she suffered were suspected to be due to a glioma, or brain cancer. But after the brain biopsy, she began to have paralysis on her left side and signs of confusion. The lesions in her brain continued to grow.

Finally, a doctor suggested that the woman might have a brain-eating amoeba. Unfortunately, it was too late. She experienced bleeding in the brain and lapsed into a coma. Her family took her off life support. After her death, it was determined that *Balamuthia mandrillaris* was indeed to blame. Quicker diagnosis and proper treatment might have saved her, but *Balamuthia mandrillaris* is notoriously difficult to detect compared to *Naegleria fowleri*.

Acanthamoeba

Yet another parasite that ravages the brain is the *Acanthamoeba*. This organism can live almost anywhere, so it's nearly impossible to avoid it, but most people who come into contact with it never get sick. That wasn't the case for nine-year-old Chris, an active, athletic youngster.

Chris's parents became concerned when he started to seem clumsy and slow, which was unusual for the boy. A few days later, Chris seemed dazed and began having cognitive difficulties and trouble concentrating. He wasn't hungry, which was very unusual. When his mother checked his temperature, it was 103°F.

Eventually, Chris was taken to the ER, where doctors performed all the standard tests, finding that his spinal fluid was abnormal. That's when the hospital's neurologist began to suspect that a virus was attacking Chris's body, so the boy was given antiviral drugs.

Instead of improving, Chris got worse. He began having seizures. An MRI found encephalitis—a dangerous inflammation of the brain that pushes the brain against the skull—but what was causing it? The doctors didn't know. But they determined that Chris was no longer able to breathe on his own, so they put him in a medically induced coma and on a ventilator, with no prediction of when—or even if—he would ever come out of it.

Fortunately, Chris responded to an experimental steroid treatment and began to regain consciousness and breathe on his own. Eventually, he opened his eyes and saw his anxious parents. Then, an infectious disease specialist performed another test and found that the boy was infected with the *Acanthamoeba* parasite. Once the cause was known, Chris was back on his feet after six more weeks of rehabilitation and had recovered his neural functions and speech.

Acanthamoeba is a difficult organism to avoid—it lives almost everywhere in the environment, including ponds, swimming pools, and air conditioning units. There's no telling where or how Chris acquired the infection or why he was hit so hard by it. *Acanthamoeba* is better known as an infection of the eye when someone wears or sleeps in unsanitary contact lenses. Even then, it can devour the eye instead of the brain.

Chapter 4

Beware of Deadly Spiders

*M*ost spiders are harmless. They can be a nuisance, and many people are death-ly afraid of them, a condition called "arachnophobia." Those people have a point, though. There are spiders around the world that are far from harmless. Rather than just taking these outdoors and letting them go, you should avoid them at all costs—they can maim or even kill.

A New Threat

Mexican scientists have recently discovered, not far from Mexico City, a previously unknown venomous spider that they call *Loxosceles Tenochtitlan*. The eight-legged beast is a brown or tan color and doesn't look particularly threatening, but its bite can cause lesions of dying tissue, which can be over 15 inches long, in human flesh. The bites can take months to heal and leave permanent scars. The spider's bite is particularly dangerous to children, as the venom can enter their bloodstream and destroy red blood cells. The female of the species is twice as venomous as the males.

It belongs to a group of other venomous spiders that can rot human flesh with a single bite. At first, the new spider was mistaken for another *Loxosceles* spider, and it was thought to have been imported into the area in shipments of ornamental plants. Then it turned out that it was completely unknown to science, though it is related to other arachnids known as violin spiders, recluse spiders, and reapers.

What makes these spiders more likely to bite people is that they hide in homes under furniture or clothes. Merely sitting on the sofa can result in a nasty and dangerous surprise! Our houses contain the right temperature and humidity for the spiders to survive and thrive. Other places that they inhabit are warehouses and trash piles, where they can encounter cockroaches and other tasty bugs to eat. If they feel threatened, they can attack.

The Deadly Black Widow and Its Relative

Everyone knows to beware of the glossy black spider with the bright-red hourglass shape on its abdomen—the black widow. Long considered the most deadly of spiders, the black widow's bite doesn't usually cause death but can cause severe illness. There are five different species of black widow spiders in North America, some of which have different shapes for their showy red warning signs. As the name suggests, the female of the species is more dangerous than the male.

In the early 1900s, the treatments for black widow spider bites could be as deadly as the insects themselves. Treatments included alcohol (taken internally), strychnine, cocaine, ammonia, and morphine. It was not altogether clear whether one man, who was bitten by a spider in an outhouse, died of the bite or the doctors' remedies. These days, anti-venom is available that can alleviate the suffering if the bite is recognized early enough. Actually, though, doctors still use opioids to combat the great pain that black widow spider bites can cause.

More recently, Albania has experienced a resurgence in black widow spiders, some of which have proved deadly. A 17-year-old boy and a 27-year-old woman, both previously perfectly healthy, died after being attacked by the spiders, and officials suspect that the black widows are invading southern Europe, perhaps coming in on ships since trade has increased in countries that border the Adriatic Sea. There have been other reports of bites and more deaths as well. Doses of the antidote were sent from nearby Croatia as hundreds of people flooded emergency rooms to have their spider bites examined.

Even when they're not fatal, black widow bites can cause excruciating pain and even cardiac complications. A young US soldier was bitten on the penis while using a portable toilet at a training site in Texas. In addition to pain at the site of the bite and surrounding areas, he experienced weakness, severe abdominal and back pain, headaches, and nausea. He became pale, sweaty, and wracked with anxiety. His pain worsened instead of lessening in the next few days and began to affect his heart and other body systems as well. Transferred to the intensive care unit, he was at last treated with antivenom, which worked to alleviate his symptoms within five days.

Pam, a 56-year-old woman from North Carolina, was not so fortunate. Her black widow spider bite in her upper right arm proved fatal after only one day, despite the fact that she was cared for in the ICU. Pam was gardening when she first noticed the bite. She experienced increasing pain and a raised, bruised-looking area where the spider had bitten her. Through the night, her symptoms progressed to greater pain, nausea, and vomiting. The next afternoon, she was transported to the emergency room with one of the EMTs supporting her breathing. She was later admitted to the ICU. Pam's skin became dusky, bluish, and cold to the touch, and she was unresponsive. Doctors found a lesion nearly ten inches long on her inner arm and could not get a blood pressure reading. Her kidneys seemed to be involved as well. Her brother and twin teenagers rushed to her bedside. In just over 24 hours after she was bitten, Pam died of septic shock caused by the neurotoxins in the spider's venom.

The False Widow

Carl, a 26-year-old lab technician in the UK, suffered a bite from the black widow's relative, called the noble false widow. One day he awoke with a red sore on his left bicep, which featured distressing pus-filled blisters. He went to an urgent care center to have it checked out. The doctors were clueless. They simply bandaged the area. Next, the wound became infected. At that time, it was only three-quarters of an inch in diameter, but the site was dark red with a ragged outline and rapidly became a foul-smelling pustule.

When it became more and more painful and Carl became shaky, feverish, and sweaty, he realized that he was really ill, left work, and went to the emergency room. The doctors didn't know what the problem was, but they tested him for everything from tuberculosis to skin cancer. None of them proved to be the answer.

After five months, the pus-filled wound still wasn't healing despite the doctors' efforts and prescriptions for three different antibiotic drugs. At last, the physicians did a biopsy, cutting some tissue from the infected site.

Then Carl found his own answer when he discovered a noble false widow spider in his bathroom. A quick search of the news told him that the number of them found in the area had been increasing. Considering everything he'd been through, Carl decided to kill the spider. The noble false widow isn't as deadly as the US black widow, but it's widespread throughout the country and is often mistaken for the black widow despite the fact that it doesn't have the red hourglass marking. Still, Carl remains nervous when he goes to sleep. Another false widow may be lurking.

The Brown Recluse

Another spider almost as feared as the black widow—and related to the one recently discovered in Mexico—is the brown recluse. Its bite can be fatal or cause great harm to the human body, as barrister Jonathon from

North London found out. Ironically, he had been on vacation to dive with sharks but was felled by a much tinier attacker!

Jonathon was on a flight from Qatar to South Africa when he felt pain in his left leg. Afterward, he said he thought he might have seen a small spider running across the floor of the airplane. Two of the flight attendants screamed when they saw the spider, too. At first, the bite wasn't all that painful, so he thought no more about it. Then his leg swelled up and took on the dark colors of a severe bruise. Afraid that he might have deep vein thrombosis from sitting for hours on the long flight, Jonathon took painkillers. Colleagues said the wound looked like a spider bite and recommended that he get medical attention right away.

Soon, the pain was so excruciating that it was the worst Jonathon had ever felt. By the time he got to the hospital, his leg was so swollen that the skin was actually breaking open, turning black, and running with pus. Doctors told him that it was definitely a brown recluse spider bite and that, if he had delayed treatment, he could have lost his leg or even died. In a desperate attempt to save his life, they began cutting away the dead and dying tissue.

When the doctors removed the bandages and revealed the damage, Jonathon said that the destruction of his dying and dead leg tissue was so shocking that he felt like he was seeing a horror movie. Then came a month of treatment for the injuries caused by the spider's venom, as well as a skin graft. Eventually, Jonathon underwent three more months of treatment. His skin graft didn't take, and he faced yet another operation.

Understandably, given that he suffered the near-fatal spider bite on an airplane, Jonathon sued the airline, saying they exhibited neglect by allowing such a deadly passenger on their plane.

Another encounter with a brown recluse had more tragic consequences. An Alabama boy named Branson died from the bite he received one Sunday morning. His mother sought help right away, but within 14 hours, her young son was dead. Doctors determined that a brown recluse was the culprit, partly because the mother took photos of the wound and the spider.

Doctors said that the boy's death was caused when his flesh began dying because the toxin entered his system and ravaged his internal organs. The red blood cells had ruptured, and Branson's urine turned a dark brown. His kidneys were clogged, leading to their breakdown.

Branson's rapid death was devastating, despite the doctor's assurances that it was less likely than death from being struck by lightning. That knowledge was little consolation to the boy's family.

Still More Dangerous Spiders

The terrifying Camel Spider (actually an arachnid species called *Solifugae*) haunts the deserts of the Middle East and Afghanistan—and even India and North America—threatening disability and death to soldiers and citizens of a number of countries. While they're not venomous, strictly speaking, they feed on dead flesh, can live in cow dung, and transfer the bacteria from them to humans that they bite. Their mouth parts are tremendous jaws that can make up one-third of their body, the largest for their body size among creatures including other spiders and even horseshoe crabs. The jaws are like a scorpion's claws. Camel spiders can be as large as eight inches and run as fast as ten miles per hour, going for hours without stopping.

Case Study

Sammy, a Scottish soldier serving in Iraq, survived his encounter with a camel spider but suffered devastating injuries. More worried about IEDs than spiders, Sammy at first didn't even notice that he had been bitten—except for two puncture marks on his thigh. The wound became inflamed and sore, so the soldier went to his company's medic, who wasn't able to help. It was two weeks before Sammy got to see a doctor. She cut open the inflamed area and drained it of fluid.

The soldier had to wait nearly a month before seeing a doctor at his base in Germany. By that time, the infection was coursing through his blood and threatening his heart. Alarmed, the medical personnel placed Sammy in intensive care. Seventeen operations later, the doctors had cut away the infected muscle in his leg, leaving a large divot in his flesh. A military medical surgeon told Sammy that he was lucky that they had saved his leg—and his life. Three years later, he had recovered only 70% of his former fitness.

Deadly Spider Relatives

Scorpions are related to spiders and can cause extreme pain and even death to anyone unlucky enough to be stung by one. The deadly sting is located on the scorpion's tail, which curves over its back. They're found in hot, dry climates, such as those in tropical and subtropical regions, as well as deserts. They kill their prey—usually insects—by injecting them with powerful venom. But sometimes scorpions attack larger animals, including humans. The results can be tragic.

Case Study

Luiz, a seven-year-old Brazilian boy, became one of the thousands of victims of the Brazilian yellow scorpion while he and his family were on a camping trip. The youngster was putting his shoes on to prepare for a hiking adventure when he felt a sharp pain. The scorpion had been lurking inside his footwear.

The boy's leg immediately began to redden, and the pain increased to an excruciating level. Luiz's parents soon found the scorpion that had stung him and immediately took their son to a hospital where antivenom was available.

But it was too late for Luiz. While he was at the children's hospital, he suffered four cardiac arrests. The doctors told his parents that they would not be able to save him. The next day, however, the boy rallied a little, but he suffered three more cardiac arrests and died just two days after he was stung. Hundreds of thousands of people in Brazil suffer scorpion stings every year, but Luiz had the bad luck to encounter one of the deadliest species.

Scientists speculate that the ongoing climate crisis has led to a vast increase in the number of scorpions by providing them with the perfect environment. In addition to the outdoors, scorpions have been found in stores and homes. In Egypt, extreme weather has caused the species of fat-tailed scorpions, which are common in Northern Africa, to flee their hiding places and move to more inhabited areas, resulting in many cases of stings and deaths.

Scorpion venom produces its deadly effects by attacking the nervous system, resulting in sweating, vomiting, abdominal pain, and paralysis. The venom travels throughout the body and devastates the heart and lungs, leading to the tragic death of young Luiz. Children and pregnant women are especially susceptible to a scorpion's venomous sting and account for most of the deaths, especially if the person doesn't receive treatment within six hours.

Scorpions inhabit the American Southwest as well as South America, India, Africa, and the Middle East. In Tucson, a two-year-old boy named Dally died from a scorpion's sting. A few years later, Dally's brother Morgan also fell victim to a scorpion, though Morgan was lucky enough to survive thanks to a new treatment developed in Mexico.

The deadliest scorpions in the world include the bark scorpion, the spitting thicktail black scorpion, the yellow fat-tailed scorpion, the Brazilian yellow scorpion, the Arabian fat-tailed scorpion, and the deathstalker scorpion. Despite their lethal danger, some people even keep *deathstalker* scorpions as pets!

Chapter 5

Leishmaniasis and Other Killer Parasites

*L*eishmaniasis and its cause, the *leishmania* parasite, may not be familiar to you. In fact, you may never have heard that parasites can infect the human body. But they're organisms that can have deadly consequences when they do. Whether they enter through a wound in the skin, in your intestinal tract through food you eat, or even through your eye, parasites can disfigure, maim, and even kill.

Leishmaniasis Attacks!

Becky was walking on the beach in Costa Rica with her

dog when she felt a bite on her arm. It was a sandfly, and the itchy bump it left meant that she had just been given a flesh-eating disease—*leishmaniasis.*

After two weeks, there was still a scab on Becky's arm, and the hole continued growing for an additional two weeks. At last, she went to a doctor for a diagnosis. The next day, he called back, told her she had leishmaniasis, and recommended that she start treatment right away. But her journey with the disease had just begun.

Becky decided against the treatment available in Costa Rica—it required 60 injections and was known to cause liver and heart damage. Instead, she flew home to the UK and sought treatment there. Her doctor there heard the diagnosis and sent her immediately to the emergency room at the School of Tropical Medicine. There, the doctor insisted on taking a biopsy, and it took five days for the results to come back. They agreed that it was the parasite leishmania. All the while, though, it continued to eat through her arm.

Two different treatments were offered. Becky could spend three weeks in the hospital receiving an IV of the same chemotherapy drugs that were offered in Costa Rica, with the possibility of liver and heart damage. Or she could participate in a trial of a new German medication given orally. It came with horrible side effects, too—so bad that many people who tried it quit taking it before the trial was over. And the drug was effective against one form of leishmaniasis—a particularly dangerous one, which was what Becky had. She began the four-week trial.

The German drug wreaked havoc on Becky's immune system. While she started to feel weaker, odd lumps appeared on her arm, and her lymph nodes swelled. One lump in particular grew painful. Abscesses from a staph infection grew under her skin and had to be drained. The infection raged through her system, making her feverish and leading to complications with her heart rate and blood pressure. She also developed a large abscess at the injection site, which the doctor had to drain pus and fluid from.

Despite antibiotic treatment, Becky developed infections in her mouth and her eye. Her left arm—opposite to where the infestation started—became abscessed as well and had to be drained and stitched.

At last, Becky's treatments worked and relieved her horrific pain and weakness. She was able to return to Costa Rica and continue her work on the sloths that live there.

What Are the Facts About Leishmaniasis?

Ironically, sloths are one of the animals that transmit leishmaniasis to sandflies, which are smaller than mosquitoes, and from there to human beings. Animals, including dogs, opossums, bats, anteaters, marsupials, and rodents, are also able to carry the leishmania parasite. About 30 different species of leishmania exist that have the ability to infect animals, sandflies, and humans.

There are three varieties of the disease based on what part of the human body they invade and what tissues they attack. *Cutaneous leishmaniasis* affects the skin and soft tissues underneath the skin, leading to sores, lesions, and permanent scarring. "Volcano" sores have a distinct appearance, with raised edges and a crater in the middle. As Becky learned, *Cutaneous leishmaniasis* and its treatments can also cause heart conditions.

Mucocutaneous leishmaniasis attacks the mucous membranes such as the nose, mouth, and other important organs. Severe sores and breakdown of mucous tissues can occur, as can difficulty breathing. *Visceral leishmaniasis*, the most deadly form of the disease, targets internal organs, provoking internal bleeding, low blood count, and enlargement of the liver and spleen as well as the bone marrow.

Leishmaniasis lurks virtually everywhere except Australia, the Pacific Islands, and Antarctica. It infests settings including the tropics and subtropics, the rainforests and deserts. In the US, it's even found in Texas and Oklahoma, as well as coming in with visitors from other countries. It's difficult to estimate, but

Leishmaniasis is thought to affect up to 1.2 million people. The sandflies tend to attack and take blood meals late in the day, from dusk until dawn.

Why Don't More People Know About Leishmaniasis?

An explorer and journalist, Pip was infected with leishmaniasis while she was working in the Amazon. She has since become a tireless advocate for people suffering from the disease. Leishmaniasis is considered one of the neglected tropical diseases (NTDs) because it usually attacks people in rural areas of poorer countries and less in the developed world. Pip wants to shine a light on the disease by sharing her experiences.

When she returned from her work in the Amazon, Pip noticed a sore on her neck—a volcano sore with crusty edges around the circular lesion. It kept getting larger and larger. It was cutaneous leishmaniasis. She had two choices, doctors said—to let it remain untreated and risk the flesh-eating parasite invading her nose and face or to take the toxic chemotherapy that Becky chose. It was no contest. Pip opted for treatment, and the doctors prepared to monitor her heart and liver function. Despite being in terrific shape from kayaking on the Amazon, by the end of the three-week treatment, she was so weak she could hardly move, and her body was in tremendous pain.

She realized that she was privileged to live in a country where specialist doctors actually had treatments to offer. A friend who lived in the remote jungle of Guyana told Pip that she had contracted leishmaniasis too but had to treat it with burning cow fat placed on her skin. Other indigenous people used crushed turtle shells in an attempt to defeat the disease. Pip realized that little research had been done to discover more about leishmaniasis and possible treatments for it, despite the fact that it's the second-largest disease caused by a killer parasite. Only malaria is more widespread.

The fact that climate change is fueling the spread of leishmaniasis and that it is encroaching on southern Europe gives Pip hope that more attention will now be paid to the parasitic disease. She particularly encourages more research on how it affects children and pregnant women—most of the sufferers who have been studied have been military men.

Still, the lack of action on climate change and humans moving into animals' home environments, such as the Amazon, mean that the disfiguring disease will likely only expand to afflict more people. Some scientists believe that the rapid pace of global warming means that leishmaniasis and other neglected tropical diseases may reach as far north as southern Canada within a few decades, exposing almost 27 million people to the disease. And while vaccines may be developed, Americans' experience fighting the COVID-19 vaccine means that any vaccine might not be widely adopted.

More Cases of Leishmaniasis

As Pip noted, *leishmaniasis* is increasingly invading the developed world, and effective treatments are not available for most sufferers. One case in north Texas illustrates this.

Case Studies

A 65-year-old man went to a dermatology clinic with three untreated volcano crater sores on his left shoulder, telling doctors that they had been there for months without healing. At first, the lesions were thought to be cancerous, but they were biopsied and revealed to indeed be leishmaniasis.

The man decided not to try the toxic treatments that Becky and Pip had undergone. Three weeks after his diagnosis, he opted instead for localized cryotherapy. After a single session of the high-tech sub-zero treatment, the sores disappeared, never to return. The side effects of *Cryotherapy leishmaniasis* are minimal, mostly discoloration of the skin, and the treatment costs are minimal compared to the more common and dangerous therapies. But, obviously, cryotherapy with liquid nitrogen is available only to a select few patients.

Patients in Pakistan had very different experiences. Amina, age two, and Asma, age three, both fell victim to *Cutaneous leishmaniasis*. Amina had a large lesion on her cheek that became infected. After seven months, it was still crusted and filled with pus. Her parents had to take her every day to a clinic 30 miles away to have the wound cleaned and dressed. Then Asma caught the disease. Their father, Raheem, found that he had lesions as well, though they resolved with some scarring.

The red area on Asma's face was also diagnosed as leishmaniasis, but she had to wait two months to begin treatment because the public clinic was so busy. Her family took her to a private clinic instead. Despite the expensive injections—which were not always available—Asma's lesion continued to grow larger over the next six weeks. At last, the treatment worked, but Asma was left with a large, deep scar. In Pakistan, the stigma surrounding facial scars makes it difficult for a girl to find a marriage partner. Plastic surgery is expensive, and it's not available except in large cities.

Idrees, a ten-year-old also from Pakistan, is another victim of the dreaded disease. The two cutaneous leishmaniasis lesions on his nose and a smaller one on his leg persisted for two years while he tried various home remedies. They only made the lesions worse. The sores turned crusty and pus-filled when they became infected. It took two years for him to be diagnosed. He must travel for 45 minutes with his older brother every day to get his medication and his dressings changed.

Idrees is terribly embarrassed by the lesion on his nose. It's made him so shy that he wears a face mask every time he goes out. Because of it, he stopped going to school when the other children bullied him—even threatening to punch him in his damaged nose. Idrees says he will return once he is healed, after he finishes his treatments.

Cases of leishmaniasis in the US are often dismissed by American doctors. Laura, a mother who was visiting Florida, and her family of five contracted the disease at the beach. They thought that they had been bitten by sand fleas, but it was actually sandflies that carried the flesh-eating parasite. The bites turned red and hard, then split open and became crusty and filled with thick, yellowish pus. Laura did research online and suspected that she and her family had leishmaniasis.

Doctors refused to believe her. They tested the family's scabby, pus-filled lesions for fungus and bacteria, pronounced them to be the common skin condition eczema, and prescribed steroid creams. The treatment may have actually made the infection worse by interfering with the family's immune system. But the parasite had been injected by the sandflies directly into the bloodstream, where it hid from tests that proved inconclusive. Eventually, Laura and her family fought off the infection, but the outcome would have been much different—even fatal—if they had caught the *Visceral* variant of leishmaniasis, which attacks the body's internal systems.

Five children, ages 2–11—refugees from the war in Syria—arrived in Beirut, Lebanon. After up to six months, they were suffering from fever, distended abdomens, and liver involvement. *Visceral leishmaniasis* was not at first suspected. They were instead diagnosed with leukemia and given treatments of steroids and blood transfusions, which would have been appropriate for leukemia but did nothing for their actual disease.

Five months later, when the children were reevaluated at a better hospital, they had terribly painful bone marrow biopsies and were correctly diagnosed with *Visceral leishmaniasis*. By that time, it had spread throughout their bodily systems. They received appropriate drug treatment after the diagnosis, but it was too late. The delay in diagnosis meant that their disease had reached an advanced, incurable state. The treatment wasn't effective, and all the children died. Doctors said they hoped that the children's cases would make other medical facilities more aware of the presence of *Visceral leishmaniasis* in the Middle East and lead to more rapid, potentially life-saving treatment.

The fact that a 42-year-old man in Italy was admitted in a timely manner to a state-of-the-art hospital was likely the reason that he made a miraculous recovery from *Visceral leishmaniasis*. Like the Syrian children, the Italian man suffered from a persistent fever and liver involvement when he was admitted, as well as fatigue and throat pain. While he waited for his test results, which took a week, he received antibiotics and immunosuppressive treatment, which had no effect at all—except to weaken his immune response. His fever and liver deterioration continued. Finally, a bone marrow biopsy revealed *Visceral leishmaniasis*, and the inappropriate treatments were discontinued. The patient survived against the odds.

A 20-year-old man in Nepal likewise survived a struggle with *Visceral leishmaniasis*. He lived in a house made of stone, wood, and mud in the hill country. The cattle shed in the yard bred flies, including sandflies. He had been experiencing symptoms for six months before he was diagnosed and treated. Up until that time, he had only received aspirin and vitamins in an attempt to treat the disease. Fever and chills had progressed to generalized weakness and a loss of appetite. Eventually, he developed a rash all over his body. After two weeks in a private hospital, the man was transferred to a government hospital. But his symptoms progressed to include abdominal pain over the next two weeks. He left the hospital despite the doctors telling him he needed to stay. Returning home, he treated his disease with ineffective natural remedies.

When his symptoms kept growing, the man again entered a private hospital. At last, a bone marrow biopsy was done. It revealed *Visceral leishmaniasis*, which explained all his symptoms, pain, and gradual decline. Again, he was transferred to a government hospital. His liver and spleen had grown to extreme proportions and caused hemorrhages in the skin above them.

After three weeks of appropriate treatment and one week of follow-up, his symptoms eased up. The severity of his *leishmaniasis* was likely caused by the delay in obtaining a diagnosis and his refusal to receive appropriate treatment when he first fell ill.

Another Killer Parasite

The only parasite that causes more disease and death than leishmaniasis is malaria. It's been around since at least the sixth century B.C. And it's responsible for a million deaths a year, despite the fact that there are now treatments and preventives for it. Most of the deaths occur in Africa, especially among children under five years old. Malaria is spread by the bites of mosquitoes that are infected with the parasite. It infects and bursts the red blood cells so that the victim's blood cannot carry oxygen to the tissues. Cellular debris blocks the blood vessels, leading to severe pain and tissue death due to a lack of oxygen.

Malaria

Malaria is bad enough when it infects the body. But when the parasite affects the brain, the results are all too often fatal. The infected person usually goes into an irreversible coma, suffers organ failure, and dies. But a few miraculous cases have occurred where someone has actually survived.

Case Studies

Jessica was one such person. She was working in the African country of Liberia. Two weeks after a visit to a small rural village, she began to notice the telltale symptoms of malaria—fever, chills, and dehydration. Soon, she wasn't able to either walk or lift her head. At first, though, she tested negative for malaria.

When her symptoms worsened, she returned to the doctor and was diagnosed with a serious parasitic infection. Despite her agonizing pain, she was sent home. She went to sleep. But she didn't wake up. She went into a coma from which no one could rouse her.

The parasite had destroyed blood vessels when it invaded blood cells. The blocked blood vessels had caused her brain to swell, pressing against the hard bones of her skull. A friend found her unconscious and got help to take Jessica to the emergency room.

Two days later, she woke up but was unable to form words and suffered from other symptoms of brain involvement such as confusion, severe head pain, and disorientation. She needed someone at her bedside around the clock. Eventually, she was evacuated to Paris because the Liberian clinic wasn't equipped to handle Jessica's severe case of malaria. In Paris, she got more effective treatment.

But the effects of malaria persisted. Jessica suffered from severe anemia, and the brain swelling she endured had pressed her optic nerve and caused partial blindness. There was no hope that the doctor could help her regain her eyesight. Later, her vision would slowly begin to return. She had survived cerebral malaria, the most deadly version of the appalling disease.

Despite the fact that malaria is most common in Africa, a four-year-old child in Italy was stricken with cerebral malaria and died from it. Officials had thought that the disease had been completely eradicated from the country, but the little girl's ordeal proved that wasn't true. A high fever meant that she had to be transported to a nearby hospital. When she fell into a coma, she was transferred to another hospital where some of the doctors had more experience with tropical medicine. Early the next morning, she was dead.

Italy had not had a case of malaria since 1970. Every time someone came down with it, they proved to be a traveler from another country. The little girl, however, had never traveled abroad. Her only travel had been to a resort northeast of Venice. The vacation fit with the incubation period for malaria, so it was likely that the parasite entered her body while she was there. Again, climate change may have caused a resurgence in the marshy coastal areas where mosquitoes breed. If the girl had been a resident of sub-Saharan Africa, she would have been only one of the 3,000 people—mostly children—who die there of malaria every day.

Halima, a three-year-old Kenyan girl, beat the odds. After two days of a high fever, although she had been treated with aspirin, she suffered convulsions before her body went limp, and her sister was unable to wake her. The family took her to a hospital that was four hours away.

When she arrived at the hospital, Halima had another convulsion, a common symptom of cerebral malaria. The doctors gave her a drug meant to treat the convulsions. But they were only a symptom. Cerebral malaria was still ravaging Halima's brain, attaching itself to the circulatory vessels.

Fifteen hours of treatment restored Halima's brain function, although she was left with weakness on her left side and a limp—a relatively mild deficit. Many children who suffer from cerebral malaria experience impairments in brain functions such as memory and attention within three to seven years. Halima's disease, despite what she went through, was deemed to be a relatively minor case.

It's doubtful that Halima's family agrees.

Chapter 6

Flesh-Eating STIs

*I*t's frightening to think how easy it is to get a disease from pursuing one of the most meaningful and enjoyable human activities. Sexually transmitted infections (STIs) are common around the world, and despite campaigns to eliminate them and treatments that are now available, they continue to spread. And as if sexually transmitted infections weren't bad enough, there are ones that can actually destroy flesh! One is a disease that has ravaged millions of people for over 500 years, and the other is one that has only recently been discovered. *Syphilis* has caused untold misery, and *donovanosis* is threatening to do the same.

Syphilis Through the Ages

Syphilis is a disease with a long and terrible history. Since it was first described around 1500 AD, syphilis has remained a mystery in many ways. Legend has it that syphilis first came to be when a Spanish prostitute had sex with a leper. However it arose, the disease has a long and gruesome history. Many historical figures are supposed to have had syphilis, though of course this can no longer be proved. Henry VIII is the most famous—certainly he had every opportunity to catch it and may even have died from it. Ivan the Terrible is another possible victim. Some people believe that his famously cruel behavior was a consequence of this illness. Famous writers and artists—and famous lover Casanova—have suffered from syphilis.

Because the social stigma of having syphilis is so great, it's also been called by other names—primarily "the pox" or "the great pox," which also referred to other STIs such as gonorrhea and pubic lice. People in France called it the "English pox," while people in England called it the "French pox" or the "French disease." Depending on which country was being slandered, it was also called the "Polish disease" and the "German disease." It's also been known as the "Spanish disease" and even the "Christian disease," perhaps because Columbus and other Christian explorers and missionaries brought it to the New World. On the other hand, some people believe that Columbus and his sailors brought syphilis from the Americas back to Europe.

What Syphilis Does to the Body

Wherever it came from, syphilis is a notorious killer and maimer that is spread by any kind of sexual contact, primarily through the mucous membranes or broken skin. The first sign of syphilis is usually one or more open sores called "chancres." It appears on the site where the infection entered the body—usually the genitals. If syphilis is treated promptly and properly, it goes away and causes no further harm.

But if the first stage of syphilis is ignored, it progresses to the second and third stages—"secondary" and "tertiary" syphilis. Why would anyone ignore it? Having syphilis still carries a stigma attached to it. Also, people who are in denial about having the disease can ignore the early symptoms since they generally go away within three to six weeks.

Secondary syphilis appears a few weeks after that. It appears as a rash over the whole body—even the palms of the hands. It's usually not itchy, but there may also be wart-like sores in the mouth or on the genitals. The rash may appear at any time up to a year and can be accompanied by muscle aches, fever, swollen lymph nodes, and a sore throat. After that, the infection goes dormant for years but doesn't go away. It's merely hidden.

It's during tertiary syphilis that the disease does severe damage to the body. If you don't get treatment, you may enter the late stage, which comes with a variety of nasty complications. Syphilis can damage the brain, nerves, eyes, heart, blood vessels, liver, nervous system, eyes, bones, and joints many years after the original, untreated infection. For some people, the bridge of the nose collapses, leaving it deformed. Or the skin and flesh of the nose can be destroyed entirely.

Let's take a look at what tertiary syphilis can do.

A Case of Tertiary Syphilis

A 20-year-old woman came to the dermatology clinic of a hospital with a reddened skin lesion on her right shoulder blade after living with it for nine months. Over the next three months, it grew and formed an ulcer with a thick lump in the middle of it. Antibiotics and even surgical treatment had no effect. The lump developed a blistered appearance and continued growing, with the skin around one edge deteriorating.

Syphilis is known as the "great imitator" because its symptoms are so often mistaken for other conditions. Doctors tested the woman for various bacterial, viral, and fungal infections, including hepatitis B and C and HIV, but not syphilis. They took a piece of her lesion for examination and found her big lesion swollen, scabbed, inflamed, and oozing.

Naturally, the doctors took the patient's history. She reported having had mouth sores for the last five years and a painless lesion on her genitals that went away on its own. She also said she had pain in her right hip and leg. She claimed that she had been having sex with her partner for three years and that neither one of them had other partners. But she noted that he had also had a painless lesion on his penis, which disappeared without leaving a scar.

By this time, the sore on her shoulder blade had grown even larger and more grotesque. It had red, crusty edges and a number of yellow, ulcerated spots within the larger lesion. The lump in the middle of it was open and bright red. Also, she developed swollen skin and tissue on her scalp, along with greasy yellow scales. There was also an eroded area on her lower lip.

Still, syphilis was not suspected. More tests revealed systemic vasculitis and inflammation in both eyes. A CAT scan showed that the woman's bones were damaged and swollen. This time, doctors thought she might be suffering from cancer.

At last, a test proved positive for syphilis in both the woman and her partner. Her treatment changed dramatically. A neurological examination and a consultation with an orthopedic specialist were ordered. The tertiary syphilis had invaded her skin, central nervous system, eyes, and bones. She finally received treatment with penicillin, the standard drug used since it was discovered that it cured syphilis when it was started early.

Although the woman's condition improved, she was left with extensive scarring on her shoulder blade and a tumor on her right collarbone.

The Newest STI

Most people have never heard of donovanosis, but it's the latest STI to be reported—and it's a flesh-eating menace. The bacterial infection produces bleeding ulcers on the genitals and is spread by sexual contact of any kind, including oral sex. In rare cases, it can even be spread by skin-to-skin, nonsexual contact. And it can be transmitted from an infected mother to her baby as it goes through the birth canal.

What Does Donovanosis Do to the Human Body?

Since so few people have heard of donovanosis, they may not realize they have it until it shows up with the typical sores in the genital area. These sores signal the onset of a potentially disfiguring disease.

Symptoms of the STI

If the donovanosis bacteria invade your body, it will progressively destroy your genital tissue and anus, if that's where the infection entered your body. You will get bulging red bumps in your genital area that grow larger the longer you avoid treatment. The many blood vessels in the area break down. The skin on the red bumps wears away, and they begin bleeding. The lesions are often described as "beefy red" in color because of their bloody appearance.

Numerous ulcers in your genital area are another sign that you're infected. Your skin will be damaged, and your genitals will lose their color. Diagnosis may be difficult, though, as the symptoms can be mistaken for other diseases such as chancroid, cutaneous amebiasis, lymphogranuloma, or even cancer. The doctor will have to scrape the base of your ulcers to get tissue to test.

Other types of symptoms are possible. In addition to or instead of the bleeding lesions, you may have drier ones with irregular edges and a dry texture. Some people even describe these as having a "walnut-like" appearance. Necrotic lesions are deep and cause tissue destruction—flesh-eating. And then there are ones that produce scars. In women, the scarring caused by long-lasting ulcers can appear like the aftereffects of elephantiasis (which we'll discuss in Chapter 8). Don't get complacent if your symptoms seem to disappear. The bloody ulcers will grow back even after they seem to have gone away.

The early signs of the infection are not usually painful, which may lead some people to ignore them. But they should be taken seriously. Lasting complications are possible if the infection isn't treated in time or is undertreated—for example, if you quit taking the prescribed antibiotics sooner than you should according to the doctor's prescription.

Not following the doctor's orders leads to a number of possible complications. In addition to inflammation, tissue damage, and scarring, the donovanosis infection can spread to your pelvis, bones, and internal organs. Damage to the mouth, genitals, urethra, and bowels can occur. If left untreated, the disease can even lead to cancer.

Who's at Risk?

Donovanosis is more common in subtropical and tropical countries and regions, including Brazil and the Caribbean, but it's invading the US and UK as well.

Anyone who has sex is at risk, but right now the infection is most often found in people between the ages of 20 and 40.

One of the many hazards of donovanosis is that the symptoms only start appearing one to four months after you get the infection, so it's quite possible to pass it on to others during that time. If a partner has developed donovanosis in the last 60 days, you should see a doctor, even if you don't have symptoms yourself.

And a quick shot of penicillin is not an easy cure for the disease. The doctor will treat you with three weeks or more of antibiotics and will want to follow up with you to make sure no more symptoms have appeared. You could have a relapse within six to eighteen months after the sores appear to have healed. And you could need surgery to remove the scar tissue that the infection can leave.

The best way to prevent getting infected with donovanosis is to always use a barrier method of protection, such as a condom—one that fits well and stays on throughout the sex act. Not using protection is the most dangerous habit that can lead to catching donovanosis. As with most STIs, there are other risk factors that make it more likely you'll get infected. Having multiple sex partners is an obvious one, along with not being tested for diseases if you do. Traveling to a region where donovanosis lurks can also be a risk factor. And poor hygiene will make the infection worse.

Ironically, the COVID-19 pandemic led to a lower rate of donovanosis because so many people were isolating, quarantined, or observing social distancing.

Cases of Donovanosis

Since it has been so recently publicized, donovanosis cases are rare and often misdiagnosed. There has been a report from the UK on a young woman (somewhere between 15 and 25 years old) who came down with the infection. The pharmacist who uncovered the report warned that the STI could cause the genitals to literally rot away. The cases below proved that it did.

That grim prediction was borne out by a case in India. A 50-year-old woman came to an outpatient clinic with an ulcerated sore on her genital area that she had had for five years. It was painless, but it bled when touched. She reported that it had started as a small skin lesion that later became ulcerated and covered her entire vulva. She also had swollen lymph nodes in her groin. Donovanosis was diagnosed after a tissue smear.

Unfortunately, because the woman waited so long to have her bleeding ulcer examined, it didn't respond to antibiotics. The doctors took tissue samples from both the woman's ulcer and lymph nodes. They found cancer, and she was referred to a specialist cancer center.

The infection had continued for so long that surgical removal of her entire genital area and her lymph nodes was required.

An 18-year-old in India also suffered from donovanosis. She had a history of unprotected sex and developed a nodule on her genitals that kept growing larger over the course of eight months. When the egg-shaped lump became a bleeding ulcer, she sought treatment. That too increased in size, and a lymph node in the area was visibly ulcerated as well. The lymph node also bled when touched.

Doctors took a biopsy specimen from the edge of the genital ulcer, along with smears from the ulcer and the oozing lymph node. Later, an even deeper biopsy was needed. Donovanosis was diagnosed, but the lymph node showed no sign of cancer.

The young woman was given the standard antibiotic treatment, with absolutely no improvement. She underwent surgical removal of her genital region and dissection of her lymph node.

Chapter 7

Deadly Plant Infections

*P*lants are pretty. Some of them are useful as well. Plants provide a great portion of the world's nutrition. But when plants go bad, the consequences for humans can be disastrous.

Watch Out for Thorns!

Everyone knows that a prick from a rose's thorn can be annoying and painful. But there are thorns that can transmit deadly diseases. There are also plants like fungi and yeast that can afflict you with dire conditions.

Case Studies

Mycetoma is one of these flesh-eating fungi. For 15-year-old Alsadik of Sudan, it all started with the prick of an acacia thorn on the sole of his foot. He cleaned the small wound and continued playing. Within a week, he developed an infection at the site where the thorn had pierced his flesh. Like many teens, he ignored that too—until he began to develop sores.

A year later, the sores were massive, damaging his foot and spreading up his leg. Doctors diagnosed *mycetoma*, a fungus that entered his body when he pricked his foot, allowing the disease to get in.

Mycetoma is a fungal disease that can also allow bacterial infections to invade the body. There's no way to prevent it. It's present in the soil throughout Africa and has made its way into Mexico as well. The open, disfiguring sores the fungus causes predominantly affect poor people. Drugs to treat it are expensive—the treatment is four pills a day for two or three years. If the drugs are available to them at all, many people must take out loans to pay the costs. The medicines also have extreme side effects, including liver failure, which can lead to death. People who try native remedies often get secondary bacterial infections that add to the progression of the disease. *Mycetoma* has only a 27% cure rate.

After about a year, the sores on Alsadik's leg had grown into huge, gaping wounds. He finally went to the hospital and had another operation to remove dead flesh and stem the tide of infection. He left school after the surgery to clean out the massive wounds. Though he believed he was cured, the sores returned within two years. And they were worse than ever.

At last, Alsadik visited a research center where doctors were more knowledgeable about *mycetoma*. They tried a number of treatments and operated on Alsadik's leg a total of seven times. But the infection proved too strong for the drugs and surgeries to cure. It was simply too advanced. Alsadik was in so much agony that he had to take painkillers just to walk. He decided that the only solution was to have his leg amputated at the knee. Despite the amputation, Alsadik knows that he is not completely cured. The *mycetoma* can still recur. Nineteen years later, he was still taking treatments that would have cost $5,000 if he could afford them. Alsadik has had to rely on help from others to get the treatments. Now 34 years old, he has difficulty supporting his wife and children with no job.

In Africa, *mycetoma* is considered a "silent killer," another neglected tropical disease. The one research center that deals with the fungus hopes to find a better treatment—one that will require only one pill a week for one year. In a small village of 1,000, approximately 80 people will have *mycetoma*. They're likely to be 40 years old or younger, and one-quarter of the victims are children.

A 26-year-old Sudanese man, Mustafa, also suffers from *mycetoma*. Like Alsadik, he at first ignored a thorn in his knee. He went off to college to study accounting. But his knee was swelling, and it was difficult to get to class. The swelling was as big as a cantaloupe and oozed putrid pus and crusty black fungal spores.

Mustafa's case was typical of *mycetoma* fungal infections. Small sores appear early but disappear quickly, only to come back later, more extreme and disfiguring than ever. The fungus multiplies beneath the skin, pushing aside muscles, tendons, and even bones. Bulges form, and then lesions break the skin and discharge the spores into the environment.

The cost and side effects of the medication meant that Mustafa had to quit taking it and return to his home village. There, a local healer treated the lesions with a paste of battery acid, which was excruciatingly painful and did nothing to stop the spread of the disease. It was cheaper than the treatment at the research center but held no hope of a cure. Mustafa returned to college and the research center in Khartoum, but by then *mycetoma* had dug out cavities in his flesh and bones. The smell was so putrid and embarrassing that he again had to quit his classes and leave college. Another traditional healer prescribed herbal potions, but the disease only got worse.

Like Alsadik, Mustafa had his leg amputated above the knee. But that wasn't the end of his suffering. Fungus remained in his body, spreading to his groin and then even to his lungs. He tried another drug, this one imported from India, but took only two pills a day instead of the prescribed four in order to keep the cost down. Doctors at the research center gave up, saying they could do nothing more for Mustafa.

More Flesh-Eating Plant Diseases

A fungus called *Chondrostereum purpureum* causes a disease, usually in roses, called silver leaf disease. It's spread by airborne spores and kills the plant. Unfortunately, it can also do that to human beings.

Case Studies

A 61-year-old man in India who worked with mushrooms and plant fungi started experiencing a cough, a hoarse voice, and difficulty swallowing. He was fatigued, but he lived with his symptoms for three months. He had no history of respiratory ailments or immunocompromising diseases.

The silver leaf disease was revealed when it turned out the man had a huge abscess in his neck that partly obstructed his airway. No wonder his voice had been hoarse! Doctors drained the pus from the abscess and started him on antifungal medications every day for two months.

The man healed, and the disease hasn't returned. But scientists are concerned about what his experience means for the possibility of other plant fungi or diseases infecting humans.

One fungus that has proven deadly to people who encounter it is *Apophysomyces*, which produces a flesh-eating disease called mucormycosis. Necrotizing lesions occur when the fungus enters the skin, often through traumatic injury. The fatality rate is significantly high.

Thirteen cases of the flesh-eating fungus resulted in the wake of a tornado that struck Joplin, MO. One 61-year-old woman had no traumatic injuries but most likely caught the fungus when the soil around town was disturbed and flung through the air. Ten months after the tornado, she came to the local hospital with a fever and a necrotizing infection in her right arm. It was progressing rapidly, eating into her flesh. Broad-spectrum antibiotics had no effect, and she underwent surgery to root out the infected tissue. The fungus had even invaded her blood vessel walls. Within two days, she required two more surgeries on her devastated flesh.

Then the woman was transferred to another hospital and admitted to the surgical intensive care unit. Yet another surgery revealed that her soft tissues, biceps, and other muscles were involved. While she remained in the hospital, the infection crept toward her chest and back and required still more surgeries. The woman developed low blood pressure and respiratory failure. Her condition continued to deteriorate, and on the seventh day since she was hospitalized, she died.

Another plant-based disease is *sporotrichosis*, also called "rose-picker's disease." This fungus may sound harmless, but while it afflicts mostly farmers, gardeners, workers at plant nurseries, and—for some reason—carpenters, it can burrow into your flesh and produce ulcerated lesions. The symptoms start out mild, but can lead to serious complications.

Sporotrichosis is found all around the world, especially in Central and South America. It lives in rose bushes, hay, moss, and the soil around these plants. The fungus can hitchhike on rose thorns and find a way into your body when they pierce your skin. There are two kinds of *sporotrichosis*: cutaneous (skin-based) and pulmonary (lung-based), which is caused when you breathe in the spores instead of pricking your skin. If you don't treat the infection, it can become permanent, so see your doctor for a skin biopsy if you think you have it. Symptoms, in addition to red or purple bumps and open sores, can include headaches, joint pain, and seizures. Skin infestations require that you take anti-fungal treatments for several months. If the infection is severe, you may have to have IV treatments, then an antifungal for up to one year. If you have pulmonary *sporotrichosis*, you may require surgery to remove infected lung tissue.

Plant Toxins

Plants can also produce toxins that are harmful to people. Any part of a plant can be toxic, including leaves, fruit, stems, and seeds. They can produce inflammation, painful skin blisters, and even blindness.

The Manchineel Plant

The manchineel plant, for example, is one in which all parts are poisonous. The sap is toxic. Water dripping from a tree that carries the sap is hazardous. Even smoke from a burning manchineel tree can cause blindness. Eating manchineel fruit results in inflammation and burning lesions around the mouth. It's also known as the Tree of Death, and its fruit is known as the Little

Apple of Death. Its toxins have even been used to create poisoned arrows.

You can find the manchineel tree in coastal areas of the southern US, as well as in Central and South America and the Caribbean. Manchineels can live on beaches and in swamps. It's very attractive, luring in plant-loving people.

One woman named Nicola had an encounter with a manchineel tree and its fruit on the Caribbean island of Tobago. On an idyllic beach, she found some green fruits that were about the size of a tangerine. They came from a large tree with silvery bark. Unwary, Nicola picked up one of the fruits, and she and a friend took a bite.

Shortly after, she noticed a sensation in her mouth that reminded her of pepper. Soon, it turned into a burning sensation and a tearing feeling that accompanied tightness in her throat. In a couple of hours, she and her friend could no longer swallow food because of the searing pain and a prominent lump in her throat. Unfortunately, water did nothing to ease the pain and burning. It took eight hours for the searing pain to go away, but the encounter left her with swollen lymph nodes. Local people were horrified that she had eaten the fruit.

The small amount of juice that Nicola swallowed had caused ulceration in her mouth and swelling in her throat. Ironically, she was a medical professional and should have known better than to bite into an unfamiliar fruit that she simply picked up on a beach. Fortunately, she and her friend escaped the potentially fatal consequences. She noted that the fruit would pose a particular danger to children, who would be attracted by its appearance, sweet smell, and taste.

Hogweed Plant

Yet another dangerous plant is the giant hogweed plant. Ironically, it's a member of the carrot family but is hardly one of its innocuous cousins. The nasty sap from anywhere on the plant can cause blisters that leave scars if it touches bare skin. And if any of the sap gets in your eyes, you can become permanently blind. Its flowers are white and pretty, like Queen Anne's lace.

The giant hogweed came from the region between the Black Sea and the Caspian Sea. It was imported to the US around the 1900s for display in decorative gardens and arboretums. But it escaped from cultivation and began to run wild in New England, the Northwest, and the mid-Atlantic states. It's even made it as far as Michigan, where officials are warning locals about its dangers and trying to eradicate it. It's so hazardous that it's illegal to sell or transport it across state lines.

Chapter 8

What's Elephantiasis?

*L*ymphatic filariasis (LF), better known as elephantiasis, is a disfiguring disease that causes your limbs—and even your genitals—to swell grotesquely. It's caused by a parasitic, thread-like worm called filaria that is spread by mosquitoes. When it gets inside you, the results are horrendous. It can lead to shame, shunning, and permanent disability. Here's a look at life with elephantiasis.

The Facts About Elephantiasis

Swollen legs, arms, breasts, and/or genitals are the hallmarks of elephantiasis. The disease got its common name because the swollen limb takes on the appearance and toughness of an elephant's skin. It's not only disfiguring but also causes pain and disability. Next to malaria, LF is the most common parasitic disease in the world, affecting around 120 million people in 72 countries, most of them in the tropics and subtropics of Asia, Africa, the Western Pacific, and parts of the Caribbean and South America (CDC, 2019). It's particularly rampant in areas with poor sanitation and poverty.

Elephantiasis is caused and spread by a tiny, thread-like roundworm that is transmitted by an infected mosquito when it takes a blood meal from a person. The worm invades the human lymph vessels, an integral part of the all-important immune system. When they're infected, the lymph nodes fill with fluid as the worms grow to adult size. This causes the exaggerated swelling of limbs, hardened and thickened skin, and nodules. Because elephantiasis attacks the lymphatic system, it makes it easier for the affected person to get even more infections. These come with their own symptoms, such as fever and severe pain.

It's incurable, but there are drug treatments for elephantiasis that can be taken once a year. The medication kills the worm larvae but does nothing to the adult filaria. If the infection involves the scrotum, surgery may be necessary to diminish the swelling. Eradicating the disease also requires eliminating the places where mosquitoes live and breed.

Living With Elephantiasis

From the time she was a child of nine in Spain, Maria had noticed her knees and legs growing larger and larger, to the point where she could no longer wear shoes. But she and her parents weren't worried—at first. By the time she should have graduated from high school, Marie was bedridden. For more than ten years, her world was restricted to her bedroom and bathroom. She dreaded the idea of going out anyway, where she would be stared at and talked about. Her family were the only people she saw.

Completely mystified, Maria's doctor posted an account of her case online, where it was seen by the manager of the Spanish office of a German medical equipment company. She connected Maria with a doctor in Germany who thought there was hope of a recovery. When insurance refused to pay for her treatment, the medical equipment company and the general public chipped in to provide the funds.

Maria arrived at a clinic in Germany, but she needed helpers to get her out of the ambulance, into the building, and to her bed. Marie had elephantiasis and could barely move. Her right calf was 62 inches in diameter. Both legs were grotesquely swollen with massive rolls of what looked like fat but were really a backup of lymph fluid. Six months after she entered the clinic, the doctors had drained 190 pounds of fluid from her legs. Her calf shrank to just over 20 inches in diameter.

Now Maria is back in her hometown. She maintains the progress she made in Germany by wearing special garments, which the medical equipment company provides, to apply pressure to her legs. The doctors hope that she can live on her own in Spain and return to Germany only occasionally for further treatment.

Rodwell, 72, lives in Guyana and was a dancer until elephantiasis struck, crippling his left leg and making it impossible for him to wear dancing shoes. Pain and swelling in his foot were the symptoms that first brought him to the ER and then to a clinic for Lymphatic filariasis when he was diagnosed.

The clinic gives out medicine to prevent the disease, but like so many others, Rodwell never thought he needed to take it. Until he contracted the disease himself, he didn't realize the danger. Because his disease was caught early, Rodwell's elephantiasis was able to be treated. Now that he knows about the dangers of *Lymphatic filariasis*, he's active in the efforts to warn others and encourage them to get help. And now that he can get his shoe back on, he's back to dancing.

Indumati lives in a part of India where nearly half the people suffer from elephantiasis. The 58-year-old widow has lived with the disease for almost 25 years. Treatment has done little to relieve the huge swelling and ugly lesions on her right leg and foot. Unable to work or walk, she has been afraid to leave her village because of the stigma and shame. She even feared visiting her children for fear that they would get the disease too and suffer like she did. Indumati was isolated and had little hope.

CASA, a non-governmental organization, started an outreach program in Indumati's village, offering treatment and education on the dangers of LF in hopes of eliminating the cycle of transmission. Simple practices like washing affected areas with soap and water and getting exercise can lessen the severity of attacks and enable sufferers to work at least a month more per year. It's helped Indumati. Her swelling has decreased, and now she doesn't hesitate to visit her grandchildren.

Algueta, who lives in Nigeria, contracted elephantiasis when she was in her teens. She knew she was ill when she became plagued with fevers and headaches and her legs began to swell rapidly. The symptoms didn't respond to ordinary medication. Algueta was shunned by the people in her village, and her family was accused of witchcraft.

Fortunately, Algueta was able to travel to the neighboring country of Burkina Faso, where she could get treatment from a new program that had been introduced. There, she received a combination of antiparasitic drugs. They cleared the parasite from Algueta's body, but her condition remained permanent. Both of her legs remain hugely swollen, with her right one as large as a tree trunk.

Edou lives in Togo, one of the countries in Africa where elephantiasis is endemic. At first, he was suddenly plagued with symptoms of fever and nausea. He went to his local village hospital, where he was treated with anti-malarial drugs and given a tetanus shot. Of course, these did no good since he wasn't infected with malaria or tetanus. Edou's condition only worsened, and his legs and genitals swelled to grotesque proportions. He was forced to give up his job as a driver and mechanic, leaving him with no way to support his wife and seven children.

When a treatment program finally reached Edou's village, he began to receive the care he needed. Drugs stopped the swelling in his legs. He needed surgery to correct the swelling of his scrotum. After he recovered from the operation, he once again began providing for his family by farming pigs.

Filariasis of the Eye

While most elephantiasis affects a person's arms and legs, it's possible for the filaria worms to invade the human eyeball as well. When that happens, it's called loa-loa, loiasis, or African eye worm. Unlike with elephantiasis, where the worms are microscopic, the filaria worms are visible as they crawl across the surface of the eyes and through the skin around them. And the loa-loa worms are transmitted not by mosquitoes but by deer flies. The disease can produce no symptoms at first, but eventually, as the worm migrates to the eyeball, the eye itches and the skin around it swells. Worst of all, the infected person has the sensation of something crawling in their eye—because that's exactly what's happening.

Case Studies

In fact, it happened to theology student Israel while he was on a missionary trip to Equatorial Guinea. The first symptom he noticed, however, had nothing to do with his eye. Israel discovered itchy, hot, red bumps on his leg, and then later, similar large bumps on his abdomen, sized and shaped like an egg. They went away on their own, so he wasn't worried.

His next symptom was a feeling of lethargy and a fever of 103 degrees Fahrenheit. Israel refused to go to the doctor, and the fever broke on its own. But he couldn't ignore it any longer when his right eye began to itch. The pain was unbearable. He asked his wife to look into his eyes. She saw what looked like an inflamed vein, but then it started moving. It was a wiggling, string-like object, and it was moving around under the outer layer of Israel's eye.

At last, Israel went to the hospital. The triage nurse couldn't see anything wrong. She thought Israel might have a condition called "delusional parasitosis," where patients think they are infected by a parasite when they really aren't. When an ER resident looked into his eye, however, she saw the same moving creature. The fact that he had been in West Africa gave her the clue she needed. Israel had been infected by the loa-loa worm. For two years, it had been living between the layers of connective tissue under his skin and feeding on his body fluids. This was what caused the annoying red bumps that erupted on his leg and abdomen—side effects of the infestation called "Calabar swellings." Eventually, the worm burrowed its way into Israel's eye.

If Israel hadn't discovered the worm in his eye, it could have stayed in his body for up to 17 years, invaded his kidneys and lungs, and caused scarring around his heart. But after two weeks of treatment with an antiparasitic drug, the worm was gone.

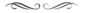

Carmen, who lived in Florida, was another victim of the parasitic worm. The filaria worm had been feeding on the nutrients in Carmen's bloodstream, causing inflammation, headaches, and extreme pain. When it was discovered in her eye, her doctor knew he must get it out as soon as possible—all of it. That proved difficult. Carmen was given a local anesthetic, and he cut into her eye in an attempt to get hold of the worm. He kept pulling and pulling, but the worm seemed to keep coming. When he got it out at last, he was looking at a worm that was nearly eight inches long. And it was lucky that it hadn't grown any longer—the filaria worm can grow up to a foot long!

Chapter 9

Killer Animal Diseases

nimals add meaning to our lives. Pets are our companions. They give us affection, provide us joy, and even give us emotional support. Wild animals help us understand the natural world and inspire us with their diversity, beauty, and power. But zoonotic diseases—ones that people get from animals—wreak havoc on the human body. Bacteria and viruses that live in animals jump species when they come in contact with humans, producing some of the most feared and destructive diseases ever known.

Bubonic Plague

You may think of the bubonic plague, also known as the Black Death, as something that only happened in the past. It certainly did, beginning in the sixth century and eventually causing the deaths of at least half of the people in Europe—some historians say even more—and who-knows-how-many in China, India, and other parts of the world. But the plague that ravaged the world throughout history has not been eliminated. In fact, there are cases of plague in Asia, Africa, and even the United States every year.

There are three forms of plague: *bubonic, pneumonic,* and *septicemic.* All can be caught by handling infected animals—usually rodents—or by being bitten by fleas from infected animals. A bacteria called *Yersinia pestis* invades the human body and devastates the body's defenses against illness.

The bubonic form of the plague is the best-known. The bacteria take up residence and multiply in the lymph nodes, causing them to swell and blacken in large nodules called "buboes"—hence the names bubonic plague and the Black Death. The bacteria then spread to other parts of the body.

Pneumonic plague occurs when the bacteria invade the lungs after being transmitted by aerosolized droplets from infected people. Other people breathe in the bacteria, and the cycle continues, passing from person to person. The disease starts with shortness of breath and progresses to chest pain, coughing, and bloody mucus with respiratory failure. This is the most contagious and devastating version of the plague. Three cases of pneumonic plague were recently found in China, causing quarantines in emergency rooms and for people who had contact with the plague victims. The government clamped down on information about the cases to prevent panic among the Chinese population, perhaps adding to the possible spread of the disease.

Septicemic plague can be an early symptom of the bubonic plague or a complication that occurs after someone already has the plague. In the septicemic plague, people experience fever, chills, weakness, pain, shock, and bleeding into the tissues of the body. The skin and other tissues of the body, particularly those of the fingers, toes, and nose, can blacken and fall off or need to be amputated. It's less well understood than the other versions of the plague, but it can certainly ruin lives.

Paul caught bubonic plague one day when his cat Charlie brought home a dead mouse. He tried to take the mouse away from the cat and scratched his finger on the cat's tooth. This seemingly ordinary occurrence would change his life.

At first, Charlie the cat seemed to be the only one affected, turning lethargic and swollen. Paul had the cat put down. Then he realized that he had a fever of 103 degrees Fahrenheit, and he was diagnosed with and treated for cat scratch fever, another zoonotic disease. Days later, he again felt worse and went to the hospital's ER. The doctors there found the telltale buboes—the sure signs of bubonic plague.

Paul was transferred to the intensive care unit and put on a ventilator when his lungs failed. Then he was transferred to another hospital. He went into a coma, which lasted 27 days. When he awoke, he had lost 30 pounds, despite the fact that his whole body was swollen.

After that, Paul's limbs developed gangrene, became black, and started dying because the infection was coursing through his entire body, ravaging his fingers and toes. A month and a half later, they had to be amputated. He had more surgeries after the amputation, and he was bedridden for a long time. Physical therapy helped, but the prosthetics he was given hurt, so he stopped using them. Paul's life changed completely because his bubonic plague turned septicemic.

Lucinda and John were also stricken with the plague. The couple, who lived in New Mexico, were visiting

New York City. One morning, they woke up feeling ill. They had chills and a fever and thought they had the flu, so they stayed in their hotel room for two days. They suspected by this time that they might have the plague. They knew that it could be spread by the rodents that lived in their southwestern environment.

The hotel they were staying at recommended a doctor in New York who specialized in travel medicine. When he saw John's lymph nodes, they were textbook buboes, and they had an answer—it was indeed bubonic plague.

The couple were given antibiotics, the standard treatment for plague, but despite this, John fell into a coma. He developed gangrene in his toes, fingernails, and even his ears as the infection coursed through his blood to his extremities. The plague in his ears and fingernails pulled back, but his feet were both amputated while he was still in the coma.

John had been ill since November, and he missed both Thanksgiving and Christmas. Lucinda helped John learn to live with his new life in a wheelchair. She believed the experience brought them closer.

Seven-year-old Sierra, who lives in Colorado, barely survived an encounter with a dead squirrel while on a family camping trip. She was trying to bury the animal when a flea jumped onto her sweatshirt and bit her on the torso. A few days later, she became ill, but the whole family—including Sierra—thought it was the flu. That is, until she began running a fever of 107 degrees and having seizures. When she stopped breathing, her parents rushed her to the hospital.

The doctors there diagnosed her with febrile seizures caused by the dangerously high fever and desperately tried to lower her body temperature with ice bags. In the meantime, they conducted blood tests and treated her with antibiotics. When Sierra finally came to, she complained of pain in her leg, in the groin area, that was so extreme that she cried out. Doctors thought she must have had an abscess but struggled to determine what kind. Since she was in septic shock with infection coursing through her bloodstream, they took her to the ICU. It was a very real possibility that Sierra might not survive.

Now in a medically induced coma, Sierra still fought to live. She was treated with specialized antibiotics. Then doctors observed the rash on her torso and realized that Sierra was suffering from the plague. After five days in the coma, she started to stabilize, and her breathing tube was removed. After 17 days, Sierra was able to go home, cured of the plague, with strict instructions to stay away from dead animals.

Hazards of House Cats

Cats make excellent pets. Kittens and cats are relatively easy to care for and delight owners with their playful antics. Bringing a kitten into your household can mean hours of enjoyment. Sharing your home with an adult cat brings soothing purrs and nighttime cuddles. But they can also mean infection and disease. From cat scratch fever to toxoplasmosis to *sporotrichosis*, cats can catch illnesses that they can pass on to their human owners.

Cat Scratch Fever

Cat scratch fever is the disease you've most likely heard of when it comes to cats and humans. Just like it sounds, cat scratch fever is transmitted from kittens (more often than adult cats) to humans via scratches, bites, and even licks. The skin becomes infected with bacteria when there's an open wound—either one caused by the kitten or one the human already has. Fleas and flea excrement can also be involved in the transmission, so outdoor cats and their owners are at greater risk.

Cats don't show any signs that they are carrying the illness, so there's no way to tell if it's lurking in their system. The first sign that you've caught the disease is a skin pustule at the site of the injury. Then, a week or two later, your lymph nodes begin to swell as your body tries to fight off the infection.

Complications of cat scratch fever are possible. These include an eye infection that inflames the optic nerve and can lead to blindness. Or you can get a systemic illness that features lesions on the skin and mucous membranes, as well as the liver, spleen, and other organs. The complications are more likely to occur if your immune system is compromised and unable to fight off the infection.

Sporotrichosis

One fungus that affects both cats and humans is *sporotrichosis*. It's a disease that cats acquire when they brush against infected plants with injured skin. Then they can transmit the disease to humans through bites or scratches. The Brazilian *sporotrichosis* fungus produces more severe infections in people than other species. Some people in South America have been affected by the disease, and it may be on its way to the US.

Cases have already been found in the UK. Veterinarians and workers in cat shelters are particularly at risk, as are cat owners. In the UK, a mother and daughter and the vet who cared for their cat developed the disease.

The two women were from Brazil and had brought

the cat with them when they immigrated from Brazil. Three years later, the cat showed symptoms—lesions on its scalp and paws. The vet did biopsies of the cat's head and chin, which is when he likely acquired the infection. While the cat appeared to get better with treatment, it died unexpectedly six months later. Just to be on the safe side, the cat was cremated, along with its bedding.

The first signs of the infectious fungus are open lesions on the skin and mucous membranes, which become red and may exude fluid and become crusty. Nodules and skin ulcers appear on the head, face, and legs. *Sporotrichosis* can also lead to respiratory symptoms such as sneezing, unpleasant nasal discharge, and difficulty breathing. Lymph nodes swell. And the lesions can even affect the cartilage and bones, the lungs, and the central nervous system. People can also get eye infections from the disease.

The disease is treatable with antifungal medication for at least a month or two after the symptoms go away. Experts recommend keeping house cats away from feral cats they might encounter outdoors.

Other Zoonoses

There are many diseases that can be transmitted from animals to humans. The flu is a common example. You may have heard of "swine flu" and "avian flu." Those involve pigs and birds being the "reservoirs," or places where the disease comes from. The flu virus mutates rapidly into a form that can infect people. Because they don't have any natural immunity to the new strain of the disease, they can get a severe or even fatal infection.

But there are many other infections that can pass from animals to people. Here are a few of the worst.

Rabies

Most people know a little something about rabies—that it's transmitted by the bite of a mad dog. They also believe that the treatment for someone who contracts rabies is a series of painful shots in the abdomen. Neither of these beliefs is entirely accurate. Let's take a look at the facts about rabies.

Rabies can result from the bite or scratch of any infected mammal, not just dogs. Bats, coyotes, foxes, skunks, raccoons, and even horses and cattle can also carry the rabies virus and are just as dangerous when they bite you. Infected bats are responsible for most rabies infections in the US. It's hard to know when a bat has bitten you, so you may not realize that you've been exposed. Rabid dogs are the most common culprits in other countries. Rabies is present everywhere in the world except Antarctica.

The virus in the animal's saliva travels up the central nervous system to the brain, which loses the ability to control breathing and heartbeat. It can only be treated after the bite, but before it reaches the brain—when it gets there, the infection is almost universally fatal. Therefore, the further the bite is away from the brain, the greater the chances of survival. There is no vaccine to prevent rabies in humans, though cats and dogs are routinely vaccinated if their owners are sensible and responsible. So, most cases of rabies are transmitted by wild animals.

It's not possible to tell if an animal is infected with rabies just by looking at it. They may be aggressive and drooling, which is the usual stereotype, but they could also be unnaturally shy, timid, or bite at imaginary objects—any unusual behavior should make you suspicious. A bat on the ground is particularly suspect.

When you have been exposed to rabies, you may start feeling like you have the flu. This is the time to seek treatment. Once the symptoms progress to acute neurological symptoms, such as delirium, hallucinations, and fear of water—which is what gives rabies its other name, hydrophobia—survival is extremely rare. If you have been exposed, or it seems likely that you have, you can get treatment. The vaccine will be given over the course of two weeks—and they're shots in the arm, not the stomach. The vaccine contains tiny amounts of dead rabies virus that encourage the body to learn to fight the disease.

Case Studies

Jeanna, a 15-year-old girl from Wisconsin, was bitten on her arm by a rabid bat. The wound didn't look serious, so her parents simply cleaned it and gave it no further thought—until three weeks later, when Jeanna began developing symptoms. The symptoms were those of an acute infection—fatigue, double vision, vomiting, and tingling at the site of the bite. By the time she reached the hospital, Jeanna couldn't talk and fell in and out of consciousness. Since the virus had already reached her brain, it was too late for the vaccine.

Desperate, Jeanna's doctors sedated her and put her into a coma in hopes that her immune system could fight off the infection—something that seemed almost impossible. It was the first time this treatment had been tried; they knew the treatment might not save her life—or, if it did, Jeanna might have permanent brain damage.

Rather than trying her on the rabies vaccine, which they knew would be ineffective, the doctors put her on a cocktail of antiviral drugs. And, when Jeanna's system seemed to be fighting off the virus, they gradually brought her out of the coma.

Against all the odds, Jeanna survived, the only person known to have done so at the time. She does still have some deficits, though. Her balance is off when she runs or walks, and she speaks more slowly than before. Her doctors think the deficits may decrease over time. She's now a passionate advocate for animals and isn't even afraid of bats.

A Virginia woman exposed to rabies after being bitten by a puppy in India, where she was on a yoga retreat, was treated with the medical protocol developed in Jeanna's case. The 65-year-old woman had washed the bite with water but took no other precautions after the puppy bit her.

Once she returned to the US, the woman began having pain in her right arm. She received painkillers at an urgent care center, but doctors did not realize that she had the viral disease. Because she had waited so long to get treatment, she may have exposed others to the virus as well.

When she did go to the hospital, she was experiencing shortness of breath, anxiety, insomnia, and difficulty swallowing water—all symptoms of rabies. She later became agitated and gasped for air. Samples sent to the CDC showed that she was indeed infected with rabies.

The medically induced coma and antiviral cocktail that eventually worked for Jeanna had no effect in this case. Two weeks after she entered the hospital, the woman died. The local health department tried to track down anyone who had had contact with her, including a medical provider that the patient had bitten, and recommended that they receive the rabies vaccine. Eventually, 72 people were advised to get vaccinated. Person-to-person infection with rabies has never been confirmed, but it was thought better to err on the side of caution.

A case in Michigan also did not have a happy ending. A 55-year-old man died of rabies 12 days after being hospitalized. After his death, CDC was able to confirm that the infection was caused by a bat, even though the man had not been exposed to one—to his relatives' knowledge—for nine months. He did have a history of trapping and fostering wild animals, however. The man sought treatment after suffering ten days of pain, increasing numbness, and weakness in his left hand and arm, indicating that the infection started there.

The hospital performed a number of tests, which showed an elevated count of white blood cells and brain abnormalities. He also experienced a lack of muscle tone in his throat, which made it easy to intubate him. His muscle weakness grew to involve his right side and his legs. The man then had respiratory failure that was thought to be related to a stroke, but was more likely caused by the rabies. Eventually, he became a quadriplegic. All the while, rabies was never considered a diagnosis, though he was tested for many other viruses. When he became completely paralyzed, comatose, and brain dead, he was taken off life support. Relatives and hospital workers received treatment because of the possibility of exposure to the patient's saliva.

Psittacosis

So far, we've discussed zoonoses that can be contracted from mammals such as bats and dogs. But bird owners have to beware, too. Psittacosis is a respiratory illness that is spread by birds—both pet birds, such as parakeets and cockatiels, and poultry, including turkeys and ducks.

Psittacosis is caused by a bacteria called *Chlamydia psittaci*. It's usually impossible to know whether a bird is infected, so it's difficult to avoid if you have regular contact with birds. It's not a common disease, but you can catch it by inhaling dust infected with the bacteria that are shed in a bird's droppings and secretions or by being bitten by a bird. The people most at risk for psittacosis are bird owners, pet store employees, poultry workers, and vets.

In most cases, psittacosis starts with what seems like an ordinary respiratory illness—fever, headache, muscle aches, and a dry cough—around 5 to 14 days after encountering the bacteria. It's hard to tell whether a bird has the disease, but they may present with a poor appetite, inflamed eyes, breathing difficulty, and diarrhea.

While psittacosis usually remains a respiratory disease, when it goes systemic, it can lead to necrotizing tissue.

Case Studies

A 63-year-old woman was admitted to the ER, suffering from painful skin lesions on both her lower legs and difficulty breathing. She had been prescribed medicine for the breathing difficulty, but that was discontinued when the skin lesions appeared two days later. They were dark purple, red, and black and extended halfway up to her calf on both legs. There were also large, bulbous, raised red areas on the surfaces of her feet. The tip of her nose turned purple and black as well. It was clear her flesh was decaying because of insufficient blood flow. The woman had previously lived an active lifestyle—she cycled and gardened. Still, both her legs deteriorated and had to be amputated.

Tests were run for a number of different bacteria and viruses that cause respiratory problems, including tuberculosis and Legionella, but they all proved negative. At last, the doctors considered psittacosis. A positive test revealed an active infection. When doctors checked the woman's history, they discovered that she had had contact with tame birds, including domesticated pigeons.

Fortunately, once the cause of her infection was known, the woman survived the multi-organ failure. After six months of rehab, she was doing well.

Toxoplasmosis

We've already seen in Chapter 2 that toxoplasmosis can hijack a brain—and that we may need to keep an eye on it regarding human brains. But toxoplasmosis can also affect wildlife—again with potential consequences for people.

Four otters in California recently died with the worst bodily lesions that researchers had ever witnessed (CNN, 2023). They were killed by a previously unknown strain of toxoplasmosis. Now it's speculated that the infection might be present in the seafood that otters eat. If so, it may be transmitted to people who eat undercooked seafood, such as oysters, crabs, clams, and mussels. But the strain that infected the otters isn't the only form of toxoplasmosis that poses a threat to humans.

Case Studies

A 64-year-old woman went to a dermatologist complaining of ulcers on her hand that wouldn't heal. They started as small, blister-like lesions but had progressed to the point that they grew large and became ulcerated. The area, which covered most of the back of her hand, turned into a crusted plaque that oozed blood and pus. It was rapidly turning into an abscess.

The doctors biopsied the wound and found a densely ulcerated surface lesion that tested positive for toxoplasmosis organisms. They diagnosed the woman's illness as "cutaneous," or skin-related, toxoplasmosis. She was likely to have caught it from her pet cat. In an acute infection like the one the woman contracted, cells are parasitized and ultimately destroyed.

Fortunately, she was responsive to anti-parasite treatment, and the ugly lesions retreated and healed.

Another victim, a 43-year-old man, suffered from skin eruptions for three years before he sought treatment. The bluish-purple skin eruptions and pitted nodules were all over his legs and feet. Lab tests revealed only an elevated count of white blood cells, indicating some kind of infection.

Doctors removed a piece of tissue and examined it, looking for diseases of the blood and bone marrow. Both the upper and deeper levels of the skin showed that there was something thick and foreign that had infiltrated the tissues. The doctors decided that it was a parasitic disease—but not one of the many that attack the human gut. They detected toxoplasma parasites in the blood.

The man recovered after several months of treatment, but he was left with extensive scarring and darkened areas of skin. Although many toxoplasmosis infections of the skin happen in patients with faulty immune systems, a number of cases, including one in a three-year-old boy, have been in people with perfectly normal immune responses. Doctors warn that toxoplasmosis should be considered when patients suffer from skin lesions that never seem to heal.

Chapter 10

Terror Diseases

With all the terrible diseases that can eat your flesh and destroy your life, you'd think that everyone would avoid them like, well, the plague. But that's not so. In fact, the plague itself has been a bioweapon since it ravaged Europe as the Black Death. Dead bodies of livestock and soldiers were thrown over the walls of besieged cities in order to infect and kill the inhabitants.

Over the years, governments and groups have seen germs as a means of warfare and terror. They've developed ways to grow and "weaponize" them. The intent isn't always to kill, though much of the time it is. When it comes to war, chemical—and, increasingly, biological—weapons do more damage by tying up personnel and vital resources than by eliminating a soldier entirely. And weaponized diseases can spread from person to person, increasing the number of fatalities from one attack. Nations, including the US and Russia, have had biochemical warfare laboratories that researched the ways that different substances could be used to incapacitate or kill.

Nowadays, international agreements forbid the development and use of biological weapons—though, of course, there are "rogue states" that do so anyway. Many people are increasingly concerned that such weapons will be used by organizations, groups, and even individuals—terrorists—rather than the military. It's not fiction, either. There have been real-life examples of people using bacteria and viruses to create fear and death.

Diseases for Bio-Terrorism

So, what diseases can be used for war or terrorist purposes? Right now, some of the ones that most concern health officials are anthrax, plague, and tularemia. All are considered Category A potential bioweapons that pose the greatest threat to national security based on the ease with which they can be spread and how lethal they are. Other infectious agents, such as parasitic worms, have been explored as well.

There are certain characteristics that make a disease particularly useful for biological war and terror. To be suitable as a weapon, a disease organism should be stable enough to survive transport and administration. For example, a germ that dies rapidly when exposed to air or sunlight is not a good choice.

Another thing to consider is how the infectious agent should be delivered. Is it something that can be released into the air? Does it have to get into a person's body through a break in the skin? Can it be added to an enemy's food or water supply? Will the person releasing the bioweapon be close enough to be affected by it as well? Does the germ become active quickly, or is there an incubation period during which the person could spread the infection to others without realizing it? What's the best way to spread the biological agent—setting off a "dirty bomb?" Spraying it from an airplane?

The release of a biological agent can be done on purpose or accidentally. The members of the Rajneesh cult in Oregon targeted local residents by poisoning a restaurant salad bar with botulism. A Soviet bioweapons facility accidentally released anthrax into its immediate environment, killing at least 64 people in a nearby city and infecting dozens of others.

The Anthrax Attacks

Speaking of anthrax, one of the most notorious bio-terror incidents in modern history occurred in 2001, when anthrax germs were sent through the mail to journalists and lawmakers' offices.

Anthrax is particularly suited to biological warfare because it's easy to find in nature or produce in a lab. It lives for a long time and can be released as a powder, aerosol, spray, or in food or water. It's invisible and has no taste or odor.

Although anthrax is usually a disease of domestic and wild animals, humans can be infected when they breathe in spores or when spores enter the body through a break in the skin. It occurs in agricultural regions around the world. It's rare in the US, though outbreaks do occur, usually affecting cattle or deer.

Cutaneous (skin-related) *anthrax* is the most common way for people to get the disease. It appears as an itchy, raised bump that can be distinguished from other sores because the center of it turns black. The sore and the surrounding lymph nodes swell. Flu-like symptoms such as fever and headaches can also appear. People can also get anthrax by eating the meat of infected animals or by inhaling anthrax spores, which is the most deadly form of the disease.

During World War II, scientists doing germ warfare experiments contaminated Gruinard Island, off the coast of Scotland, with anthrax. The bacteria-laced soil on the small island made it uninhabitable. The government paid for dead livestock and blamed sick animals that came to the island on a Greek ship. The incident was largely unremembered until 1981, when a group launched a campaign to shine a light on it. They did this by placing a bucket of soil from "Anthrax Island" at a secret Ministry of Defence laboratory and alerting the news media. In 1986, the island was decontaminated with seawater and formaldehyde until no anthrax remained.

After the terrorist attacks on 9/11, the US was on the lookout for further incidents. Tough security measures were put in place at airports and strategic targets such as military bases. No one suspected that the new threat would come in such a simple way as in small envelopes.

Anthrax Terror and Panic

In October 2001, 62-year-old photojournalist Bob Stevens checked into the ER at a hospital in Florida. The doctors thought he might be suffering from meningitis. That would have been bad enough—potentially fatal—but the doctors had no clue yet that Stevens was struggling with another killer and that it would win. Two days after he showed up at the hospital, he was finally diagnosed with anthrax. Two days after that, he was dead. Four more Americans would die before the anthrax attack was over, and more than a dozen others were sickened. So soon after the 9/11 attacks, the public was terrified. It soon became apparent that the deaths were related, though officials tried to downplay the possibility of a terror attack.

The FBI was called on to investigate. They determined that the anthrax spores were contained in letters that had been sent to journalists and lawmakers in New York and Washington, DC; the first ones were mailed from New Jersey. Several postal workers were also infected. Some of the anthrax letters also contained threatening notes that seemed to have come from Islamic terrorists.

Suspicion, however, first focused on a scientist who once worked at the Army's research institute, where stocks of anthrax were kept. He was eventually cleared. Another scientist from the institute, who had been working to develop an anthrax vaccine, then came under suspicion. He killed himself before any charges were filed, and the case was closed. There is still some doubt, however, as to whether he was actually guilty. In any case, there was no link found to any Islamic group or person.

Tularemia as an Agent of Terror

The bacterial disease tularemia has been suggested as another candidate for bioterrorism use. It's very infectious and attacks the eyes, throat, lungs, and intestines as well as the skin. And it takes as little as 10 to 50 bacteria to cause illness. Also called "rabbit fever" or "deer fly fever," tularemia can be caught from ticks and deer flies or through contact with infected animals such as rabbits, rodents, and cats.

Contaminated food and water sources are also possible ways to get the infection. Or you can inhale aerosolized droplets if, for example, a lawn mower runs over an infected animal. Contaminated food and water are also possibilities for the use of tularemia as a bioweapon, but the fact that it can also be aerosolized provides another potential way to distribute the bacteria.

The incubation period is generally three to five days but can take up to two weeks. If you get the most common form of tularemia, your lymph nodes will swell, and you'll get ulcers at the site where the bacteria entered your body or rashes that can lead to permanent scarring. In severe cases, even your brain and heart can become inflamed. It's definitely life-threatening. Tularemia can also infect the eyes and cause open sores—ulcers—on the corneas. Untreated tularemia is fatal in at least 30% of cases.

As a bioweapon, it could cause fatal cases of

pneumonia. Although tularemia can be treated with some antibiotics, it's resistant to others, and developing strains of the disease resistant to antibiotics is possible and could be devastating. Aside from weaponizing and creating an aerosolized version of tularemia, it would be possible to infect food and water supplies using the corpses of rats. Tularemia germs are easy to acquire from the environment, and it's easy to grow large quantities. It also lingers in the environment for a long time, leading to more and more infections.

It's difficult to diagnose tularemia. The first symptoms resemble flu, and an infection site isn't always noticeable, especially if the bacteria is inhaled. Also, tularemia with skin lesions can be mistaken for herpes or other infections.

Case Studies

In one case that proved particularly difficult to diagnose, a 63-year-old man came to an emergency room with symptoms of fever, disorientation, and confusion. Doctors thought he might be suffering from any number of diseases, including *sporotrichosis* and deadly strains of staph and strep.

The patient didn't report any contact with wild animals and hadn't noticed the skin lesions that appeared on his legs. When they were pointed out, he did remember seeing ticks there two weeks earlier. The skin lesions were red, raised, and inflamed, with black scabs called "eschars" in the middle of them. When doctors examined the eschars, they discovered the bacteria that causes tularemia. Because of the danger to lab personnel, the samples had to be handled with biohazard precautions.

Other victims of tularemia that were misdiagnosed include infants and young children. A six-week-old infant and a ten-year-old child both came down with rashes and ulcers, accompanied by fever. Both were originally diagnosed with herpes simplex virus, and antiviral treatment for that disease was started with no effect. The fevers continued, and multiple blisters and lesions, some with black eschars, erupted.

At last, the real diagnosis emerged when the patient histories were re-examined and parents provided information about deer fly bites. Even two weeks after the infant received antibiotics, the fever and skin lesions recurred. Eventually, the doctors were able to cure the baby of tularemia.

The ten-year-old came to the hospital after having a fever for nine days, plus skin lesions and blackened eschars on the extremities and face. An evaluation at an outpatient center had resulted in a diagnosis of chickenpox, a viral disease. But the patient had been vaccinated for chickenpox at the age of fifteen months, so that couldn't be the cause. Instead, the illness was caused by multiple fly bites while the patient was working in a livestock barn. Appropriate treatment for the bacterial tularemia infection cured the illness.

Research Programs

During World War II, Japan had a biological weapons program that focused on germs that cause plague and anthrax. They also tested salmonella, typhoid, and cholera as potential weapons. In England, a bioweapons program researched botulism and anthrax. Winston Churchill authorized the production of cattle feed laced with anthrax to be dropped on Germany. After the war, the US tested brucellosis bacteria, a disease that people can get from infected animal products, on literal guinea pigs in a mock attack and tested aerosol dispersion technology. Other simulated attacks followed. In 1969, the US renounced the use of biological weapons. By 1972, 79 nations had signed a treaty forbidding them. The treaty went into effect in 1975 (Guillemin, 2006).

Throughout recent history, bioweapons programs instituted by governments have existed. In the US and the Soviet Union, research was supposed to be directed toward finding cures for biological weapons that other countries used. Research was supposed to focus on countermeasures only.

Not that the countries trusted each other to stick to the treaties. In particular, the Soviets took advantage of a lack of verification to develop an offensive bioweapons program in the 1970s and accused the US of doing the same. Cold War tensions meant that both countries kept their programs secret. Although they were definitely involved in bioweapons research during World War II, no proof has ever surfaced of the US violating the treaties once they signed them. But once the Soviet Union collapsed, evidence of their program surfaced. Soviet scientists have revealed the extent of their program. Among the projects were antibiotic-resistant tularemia and the mass production of anthrax—tons of it.

When the Cold War ended, scientific attention turned to more global communication and cooperation. But suspicion of bioweapons research has continued. During the Gulf Wars, Iran and Iraq both used bioweapons. Nor has the suspicion regarding biological weapons research subsided. During the COVID-19 pandemic, conspiracy theorists suggested that the virus was created in a Chinese bioweapons laboratory, though scientists claim that the disease most likely developed when a respiratory virus jumped species from animals to humans.

Now that war has broken out between Russia and Ukraine, fear of bioweapons is resurfacing. Russia has accused the US of funding biological weapons research facilities in Ukraine. The US—along with nations in the European Union and the World Health Organization (WHO)—funds labs in Ukraine that work to find ways to reduce the harm that bioweapons used against them would cause. But these are hardly "secret" labs. Information about them is freely available.

China, Iran, and Syria have joined Russia in making these accusations. The US says that such claims are being used to justify Russia's actions in Ukraine and to deceive Russian citizens who don't approve of the war.

The Future of Biowar

Fear regarding bioweapons and research on them goes on. While nations like Russia and China are suspected of developing—or using—germ warfare, many people are concerned with the possibility of terrorist organizations or "lone-wolf" terrorists engaging in it. Among the reasons for this are that biological agents are easy to produce in sufficient quantities and much cheaper than other types of weapons like nuclear "dirty bombs" or missiles. People who detonate biological weapons are also more likely to be able to escape before the effects of the germs take hold, making them more difficult to apprehend.

In addition to anthrax, tularemia, and plague, smallpox is another possible weapon of terror. It's extremely contagious, spreading from person to person. Despite the fact that smallpox was supposedly completely eradicated in the environment, small amounts are kept in labs in the US and Russia just in case the disease develops again and vaccines against it need to be produced. The idea that someone might get hold of these stocks of the virus is not out of the question.

Cholera is another potential bioweapon threat. A severe and often fatal bacterial disease, cholera kills millions of people worldwide each year. It spreads through contaminated water, so spreading it via a major water source might be possible. It's been weaponized in the past, so it's possible it will be in the future too.

There is also concern about innovations in the biological sciences. With the advances that are being made in fields like gene editing and recombinant DNA, it's going to be increasingly possible to modify disease organisms to make them more infectious, more contagious, more treatment-resistant, more easily spread, and more deadly. And the technology to do that is becoming cheaper and more accessible. Even pesticide-resistant insects can possibly be developed, capable of wiping out a region's crops and causing widespread starvation.

Parasitic worms are another potential bioterror weapon. They've been responsible for many human illnesses and deaths—including ones such as schistosomiasis, trichinosis, toxoplasmosis, tapeworm infection, African sleeping sickness, strongyloides, Chagas disease, cryptosporidium, babesiosis, naegleria, leishmaniasis, loa-loa, malaria, and the various amoebas. They're particularly easily found in the environment and easily collected—cheap, available, low-tech, and likely to evade the notice of security organizations. Often, their symptoms are delayed and mimic those of other infectious agents. Diagnosis can be difficult, and treatment can be problematic.

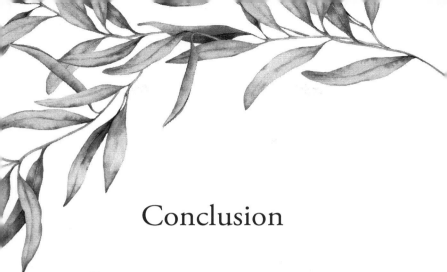

Conclusion

*S*treptococcus. *Staphylococcus. Leishmaniasis. Filaria. Klebsiella. Tularemia. Vibrio vulnificus. Acanthamoeba. Donovanosis. Loa-loa. Toxoplasmosis. Mucormycosis. Aeromonas hydrophila. Clostridium. Sporotrichosis.* Though you may not have heard of many of these organisms and diseases, you don't want to encounter any of them. They're all diseases that can change your life forever.

It's terrifying to think of your skin, flesh, heart, lungs, eyes, or brain being eaten away by something that's out of your control. But it's possible, even though it's not likely. Every day, people are infected with organisms—bacteria, viruses, fungus, worms, parasites, and amoebas—and many of those people die or suffer permanent injury.

You don't want to be one of them! You can improve your chances of staying safe and healthy if you have a front line of defense before you ever have to see a doctor. Doctors may not recognize an uncommon disease when they first see it, but you can point doctors in the right direction if you know the signs and symptoms and the ways you may have been exposed.

Necrotizing fasciitis is something doctors hope they'll never see. Even with all the training that doctors receive and the high-tech medicine available nowadays, flesh-eating diseases can sneak past health personnel with potentially fatal consequences. You can be their best assistant in identifying potential causes and starting treatment in time to save life and limb.

You need to act quickly. The speed with which these diseases progress is incredible. You can think you have only a minor infection and soon find that you're faced with something far more serious. Flesh-eating infections can require surgery to stop them from spreading, and you sure want to avoid that!

The organisms are everywhere. Innocent-looking plants, beloved pets, or even the soil in your garden can contain threats. A common mosquito bite or seemingly insignificant scratch can signal the onset. It can be the way something dangerous gets into your body.

What can you do to keep from catching one of these many infections? The best ways to stop flesh-eating bacteria from invading your body are to raise your awareness—which you've done by reading this book—and to practice good sanitation. If you can avoid situations where bacteria, viruses, fungus, and parasites flourish, you'll go a long way toward keeping yourself healthy. There may not be a way to reduce your chance of getting a flesh-eating disease to zero, but you can make it much less likely.

Reducing foreign travel to areas where these diseases lurk can help you avoid many of them. With the increase in air travel these days, someone else may bring a flesh-eating disease to where you live. But foreign travel is both enjoyable and enriching. It would be a shame to deny yourself the pleasures of traveling because of the possibility of getting a disease. But if you do travel abroad, get all the appropriate vaccinations and preventive drugs.

Insect bites transmit many of the flesh-eating diseases, so covering exposed skin and using insect repellent are advisable. If you're traveling in a place where insect-borne disease is rampant, you may even want to invest in equipment such as mosquito netting with built-in insect repellent.

Contaminated soil and water are also sources of infection. You can recycle those face masks you acquired during the COVID-19 pandemic to keep dust out of your eyes and lungs, particularly in the American Southwest. When you're at the beach, wear some kind of sandal or other foot protection. You should be careful not to drink from rivers or lakes and to wear nose plugs when you swim in them. Think about whether the water source may be polluted by run-off from nearby farms or businesses. If you're not sure, keep your nose plugs handy anyway and try not to get the water up your nose or in your mouth.

Simple hygiene is important, too. Don't stop washing your hands frequently with soap and water just because COVID-19 has pulled back a bit—and of course, after you've used the bathroom. If you get a cut or scrape, clean it thoroughly—and quickly—so bacteria don't have a chance to grow. Keep a draining or open wound bandaged with clean, dry dressings. Even a surgical wound is a potential point of entry for a dangerous disease, so make sure to keep them clean and bandaged as well, unless your doctor tells you that you can expose them to the air.

Pay particular attention to your arms and legs, especially before and after camping, hiking, or swimming. Make sure that you haven't gotten a scratch, cut, or insect bite—then keep an eye on it to make sure it's healing properly. See a doctor if you have a wound that looks infected, red, or swollen. Fast action can be needed to prevent a simple injury from turning into something much worse. Tell the doctor if you've had any insect bites or broken skin in the area where the injury is. You and your doctor are a team!

If you do have an open wound, avoid locations such as swimming pools and hot tubs—they may not be adequately sanitized—and natural bodies of water like lakes and rivers. Be particularly vigilant about warm water. The Gulf Coast is one possible site to get an illness because the water is so warm, though it's possible to get one at a cool-water beach as well. Your slim chance of getting an infection doesn't have to keep you from enjoying the pleasures of the sun and relaxation. Just lay out on the sand instead if you have a scratch or puncture on your body.

You can even help avoid potentially life-threatening diseases by paying attention to the news. If you hear about someone getting sick at a local beach, swimming hole, or water park, strike that off your list of places to visit. Come back when the danger has passed.

Don't eat produce if you don't know that it's been washed in clean, uncontaminated water. The water sprinkling system in grocery stores is meant to keep fruits and vegetables looking good for customers, not sanitize them. Wash the produce yourself when you get it home, and you should be fine! You don't have to abandon your favorite foods, either. Cook seafood like oysters and shellfish thoroughly, just in case.

Your immune system helps fight off infections and is your first line of defense. Take extra precautions if your immune system is affected by an illness like diabetes or a treatment like steroids. You don't have to encase yourself in bubble wrap and stay indoors at all times. Sensible precautions will lower your risk.

Climate change is one phenomenon that is making flesh-eating diseases more likely to spread danger. Warmer water temperatures make it more likely that bacteria can live in the water. An increase in global warming means that the danger grows greater when areas like deserts and swamps begin to take over more territory. Destruction of wildlife habitat forces animals that may carry disease—or insects that live on the animals—to invade spaces where people like to live. Think about what you can do to support organizations that address these problems. You'll help save future generations from having to deal with disease.

The efforts of organizations such as the CDC and WHO, health workers in countries around the world, well-trained medical personnel, and people like you who know what to look for will help reduce or eliminate flesh-eating diseases. Let's hope the day comes when we won't have to worry that a minor injury can be a point of entry for a serious illness.

You can help make sure that day will come! Knowing what to watch out for will save you and your loved ones from future suffering. In the meantime, you can protect yourself by taking sensible precautions. It's much better not to get a flesh-eating disease in the first place than to deal with the consequences. Let's all stay safe and healthy!

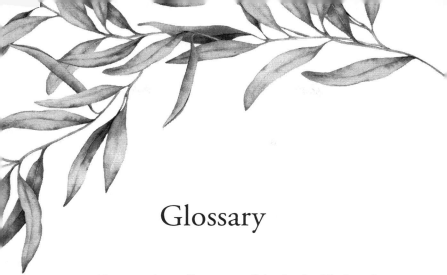

Glossary

- **Abscess:** A swollen area of the body filled with pus.
- *Acanthamoeba*: A single-celled organism that cause severe infects of the eye, nervous system, and skin.
- *Aeromonas hydrophila*: A bacteria that can cause flesh-eating disease.
- **Anthrax:** A bacterial disease that can affect the skin or lungs.
- **Babesiosis:** A disease caused by parasites, spread by ticks.
- *Balamuthia*: An amoeba that causes a severe infection in the brain.
- **Buboes:** Swollen lymph nodes.
- **Bubonic plague:** A serious bacterial infection transmitted by fleas.
- **Cellulitis:** A bacterial infection that makes the skin inflamed and swollen.
- **Cerebral:** Affecting the brain.

- **Chagas disease:** A parasitic disease transmitted to humans by insects.
- **Cholera:** A bacterial disease that is often fatal, transmitted by contaminated water.
- *Clostridium perfringens*: A bacteria that can cause flesh-eating disease.
- *Cryptosporidium*: A disease caused by parasites that can infect animals and humans.
- **Cutaneous:** Relating to the skin.
- **Donovanosis:** A sexually transmitted infection that can eat away at genital tissue.
- **Elephantiasis:** Huge swelling of the limbs or genitals caused by filaria parasites.
- **Encephalitis:** An inflammation of the brain.
- **Eczema:** A skin infection.
- **Fascia:** Connective tissue in the human body.
- **Filaria:** A parasite that causes elephantiasis.
- **Gangrene:** Death and decay of bodily tissue, often caused by bacterial infection.
- **Gas gangrene:** Rapidly spreading dead tissue in a would that gives off foul-smelling gas.
- **Granulomatous amoebic encephalitis (GAE):** An infection of the central nervous system; can also affect the skin and other organs.
- **Hyperbaric oxygen treatment:** Breathing 100% oxygen in a special chamber.
- **Inflammation:** Swelling.

- ***Klebsiella pneumoniae:*** A bacteria that can cause flesh eating disease.
- **Leishmaniasis:** A tropical disease caused by a parasite.
- **Leprosy:** A contagious, disfiguring disease that affects the skin and nerves.
- ***Loxosceles Tenochtitlan:*** A poisonous spider from Mexico.
- **Loa-loa:** An infection of the eye caused by filaria.
- **Lymphedema:** Swelling that occurs when the lymph nodes are clogged.
- **MRSA:** A respiratory disease that is resistant to antibiotics.
- **Mucocutaneous:** Affecting the mucous membranes.
- **Mycetoma:** A disease caused by fungus.
- ***Naegleria fowleri:*** Called the "brain-eating amoeba," it enters the human body through the nose.
- **Necrotizing fasciitis:** Flesh-eating disease.
- ***Ophiocordyceps:*** A fungus that can turn ants into "zombies."
- **Pneumonic plague:** Extremely contagious form of plague transmitted through the air.
- **Psittacosis:** A disease that is transmitted from birds to humans.
- **Pulmonary:** Referring to the lungs.

- **Reservoirs:** Animals where disease organisms live.
- **SARS:** A severe respiratory disease that came from birds.
- **Schistosomiasis:** an acute disease caused by parasites.
- **Septic shock:** The body's reaction to severe infection; can cause dangerously low blood pressure and organ failure.
- **Septicemia:** Blood poisoning by bacteria that moves throughout the body.
- ***Staphylococcus aureus:*** A bacteria that can cause flesh-eating disease.
- **STI:** Sexually transmitted illness.
- **Streptococcus Group A:** A bacteria that can cause flesh-eating disease.
- **Strongyloides:** A disease caused by a parasite.
- **Syphilis:** A sexually transmitted infection.
- **Systemic:** When a disease moves throughout the entire body causing damage to multiple organs.
- **Tertiary:** A disease that has progressed to a third stage.
- **Toxoplasma gondii:** An infectious parasite that can be spread by cats.
- **Tracheotomy:** A breathing hole created in the throat.

- **Trichinosis:** A parasitic disease that can affect the muscles.
- **Tularemia:** A severe bacterial infection that is transmitted by animals to humans.
- **Vibrio vulnificus:** A bacteria that can cause flesh-eating disease.
- **Visceral:** Affecting the interior organs.
- **Yersinia pestis:** The bacteria that causes plague.
- **Zoonosis:** A disease that humans can get from animals.

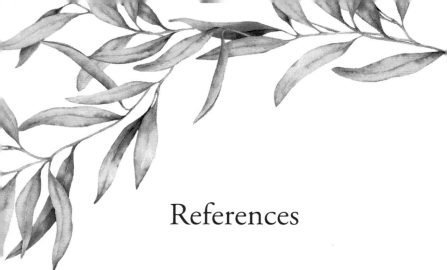

References

Acres, T. (2023, March 29). *Killer plant fungus Chondrostereum purpureum infects man in India in "world-first case."* Sky News. https://news.sky.com/story/killer-plant-fungus-chondrostereum-purpureum-infects-man-in-india-in-world-first-case-12844978#:~:text=A%20killer%20plant%20fungus%20infected

Adhikari, M., Dhakal, S., Bhattarai, S., & Rai, U. (2020). *Toxoplasmosis presenting as nonhealing cutaneous ulcer.* Case Reports in Pathology, 2020, 1–3. https://doi.org/10.1155/2020/8874800

Afshar, P. (2023, April 27). *Bacterial outbreak causes 31 infections in a Seattle hospital.* CNN. https://www.cnn.com/2023/04/27/health/seattle-klebsiella-outbreak/index.html?utm_term=1682680534207dc0f20ef17d6&utm_source=cnn_Five+Things+for+Friday%2C+April+28%2C+2023&utm_medium=email&bt_ee=9AG1S4d23VncnVkb%2F7b%2FYkLld-

5vcHhM8BrWSnQbwWd1YcND2HljTJF1SOf-
le8th0&bt_ts=1682680534210

Agrawal, M., Agarwal, A., & Arora, S. (2011). A forgotten disease reminds itself with a rare complication. *Indian Journal of Dermatology,* 56(4), 430.
https://doi.org/10.4103/0019-5154.84752

Amebic Meningitis / Encephalitis. (n.d.). Www.
dshs.texas.gov. Retrieved May 1, 2023, from
https://www.dshs.texas.gov/amebic-menin-
gitis-encephalitis#:~:text=of%20amebic%20
encephalitis.-

Andrews, L. (2023, March 24). *Rare flesh-eating parasite could jump to humans, scientists say.* Mail
Online. https://www.dailymail.co.uk/health/ar-
ticle-11899053/Rare-flesh-eating-parasite-kills-
four-otters-spread-humans.html

Archibald, B. (2012, March 19). *Under attack...
from a spider: How one soldier spent three months
in hospital after being bitten during a tour of Iraq.*
Mail Online. https://www.dailymail.co.uk/news/
article-2116970/Soldier-Sammy-O-Gorman-
hospitalised-bitten-spider-Iraq.html

Arnold, A. (2019, July 15). *What it's like to have a
flesh-eating bacteria.* The Cut. https://www.the-
cut.com/2019/07/necrotizing-fasciitis-flesh-eat-
ing-bacteria-what-its-like.html

Austin, D. (2015, August 19). Don't touch this plant;
you could go blind. *USA TODAY.* https://www.

usatoday.com/story/news/nation/2015/08/05/
blinding-plant-michigan/31125003/

Basic information | Anthrax | CDC. (2019, January
28). Cdc.gov. https://www.cdc.gov/anthrax/ba-
sics/index.html#:~:text=Anthrax%20is%20a%20
serious%20infectious

Benadjaoud, Y., & Brownstein, J. (2023, February
5). *The science behind the zombie fungus from
"The Last of Us."* ABC News. https://abcnews.
go.com/Health/science-zombie-fungus-us/sto-
ry?id=96819243#:~:text=There%20are%20
thousands%20of%20species

Benton Cooney, J. (2016, April 19). *My story of survival.* U.S. Agency for International
Development. https://medium.com/usaid-2030/
my-story-of-survival-6a127caacee4

Berezow, A. (2019, January 4). *Woman suffers terrifying death from rabies after puppy bite.*
American Council on Science and Health.
https://www.acsh.org/news/2019/01/04/wom-
an-suffers-terrifying-death-rabies-after-pup-
py-bite-13707

Bruce, S., Schroeder, T. L., Ellner, K., Rubin, H.,
Williams, T., & Wolf, J. E. (2000). Armadillo
exposure and Hansen's disease: an epidemi-
ologic survey in southern Texas. *Journal of
the American Academy of Dermatology*, 43(2

Pt 1), 223–228. https://doi.org/10.1067/mjd.2000.106368

Byington, C. L., Bender, J. R., Ampofo, K., Pavia, A. T., Korgenski, K., Daly, J. A., Christenson, J. C., & Adderson, E. E. (2008). *Tularemia with vesicular skin lesions may be mistaken for infection with herpes viruses.* Clinical Infectious Diseases. https://doi.org/10.1086/588843

CDC. (2020a, February 18). *Leishmaniasis.* Www.cdc.gov. https://www.cdc.gov/parasites/leishmaniasis/index.html#:~:text=Leishmaniasis%20is%20a%20parasitic%20disease

CDC. (2020b, May 19). *CDC - Leishmaniasis - General information - Frequently asked questions* (FAQs). Www.cdc.gov. https://www.cdc.gov/parasites/leishmaniasis/gen_info/faqs.html#:~:text=There%20are%20several%20different%20forms

CDC - Leishmaniasis - Epidemiology & risk factors. (2019, February 27). Www.cdc.gov. https://www.cdc.gov/parasites/leishmaniasis/epi.html

CDC - Lymphatic filariasis - General information - Frequently asked questions. (2019). CDC. https://www.cdc.gov/parasites/lymphaticfilariasis/gen_info/faqs.html

Centers for Disease Control. (2019). *Balamuthia.* CDC.gov. https://www.cdc.gov/parasites/balamuthia/index.html

Centers for Disease Control and Prevention. (2019). *Signs and symptoms.* CDC. https://www.cdc.gov/leprosy/symptoms/index.html

Cherney, K. (2017, August 29). *Sporotrichosis: Treatment, pictures, and rash.* Healthline. https://www.healthline.com/health/sporotrichosis#outlook

Chowdary, As., Reddy, B. S. N., & Sri, Kn. (2014). Genital donovanosis with malignant transformation: An interesting case report. *Indian Journal of Sexually Transmitted Diseases and AIDS, 35*(2), 135. https://doi.org/10.4103/0253-7184.142409

Christiansen, S. (2021, March 22). *What is Necrotizing Fasciitis?* Verywell Health. https://www.verywellhealth.com/necrotizing-fasciitis-5115254

Cliffe, B. (n.d.). *My battle with Leishmaniasis: A flesh-eating parasite - Becky Cliffe.* Beckycliffe.com. Retrieved April 17, 2023, from http://beckycliffe.com/battle-leishmaniasis-flesh-eating-parasite/

Contact lens parasite almost blinds woman | Monsters Inside Me. (2021). In YouTube. https://www.youtube.com/watch?v=Yx_v1d2x2wA

Cutaneous leishmaniasis medical care in Pakistan: Patient stories from Quetta. (2023, January 17). Médecins sans Frontières Australia | Doctors without Borders. https://msf.org.au/article/stories-patients-staff/cutaneous-leishmaniasis-medical-care-pakistan-patient-stories-quetta

Dapunt, U., Klingmann, A., Schmidmaier, G., & Moghaddam, A. (2013). *Necrotising fasciitis.* Case Reports, 2013(dec10 1), bcr2013201906–bcr2013201906. https://doi.org/10.1136/bcr-2013-201906

Duncan, J. (2018, December 30). *10 nightmarish flesh-eating pathogens that consume humans.* Listverse. https://listverse.com/2018/12/30/10-nightmarish-flesh-eating-pathogens-that-consume-humans/

Echaiz, J. F., Burnham, C.-A. D., & Bailey, T. C. (2013). A case of Apophysomyces trapeziformis necrotizing soft tissue infection. *International Journal of Infectious Diseases,* 17(12), e1240–e1242. https://doi.org/10.1016/j.ijid.2013.06.008

Eisenstadt, L. (2013, April 25). *Creature feature: African eye worm (Loa loa).* Broad Institute. https://www.broadinstitute.org/blog/creature-feature-african-eye-worm-loa-loa

Emerging transmissible sporotrichosis in cats. (2020). https://www.cdc.gov/fungal/diseases/sporotrichosis/pdf/Sporothrix-brasiliensis-Vet-508.pdf

Etienne, V. (2023, January 25). *4-year-old girl nearly dies after strep A leads to flesh-eating bacteria: "She was deteriorating."* Peoplemag. https://people.com/health/4-year-old-girl-nearly-dies-after-strep-flesh-eating-bacteria/

Father Damien . (n.d.). Www.newworldencyclopedia. org. https://www.newworldencyclopedia.org/ entry/Father_Damien

Flesh eating disease list. (2023). Study.com. https:// study.com/learn/lesson/flesh-eating-bacteria-symptoms.html

Flesh-eating bacteria patient story | Necrotizing Fasciitis. Mercy Health. (2018, November 15). Mercy Health Blog. https://blog.mercy.com/flesh-eating-bacteria-patient-story-necrotizing-fasciitis/

Frost, N. (2020, March 31). *Quarantined for life: The tragic history of US leprosy colonies.* HISTORY. https://www.history.com/news/ leprosy-colonies-us-quarantine

Gaisford, K., & Kautz, D. D. (2011). Black widow spider bite. *Dimensions of Critical Care Nursing,* 30(2), 79–86. https://doi.org/10.1097/ dcc.0b013e318205211a

Gallois, C., Hauw-Berlemont, C., Richaud, C., Bonacorsi, S., Diehl, J.-L. ., & Mainardi, J.-L. . (2015). Fatal Necrotizing Fasciitis due to necrotic toxin-producing Escherichia coli strain. *New Microbes and New Infections,* 8, 109–112. https://doi.org/10.1016/j.nmni.2015.06.003

Gamard, S. (2018, November 5). *"Flesh-eating bacteria" case: Meet the Delaware man who survived Vibrio vulnificus.* Delmarva Daily Times. https://www.delmarvanow.com/story/news/

local/delaware/2018/11/05/vibrio-vulnificus-meet-man-who-beat-flesh-eating-bacteria/1803759002/

Gaudlip, A. (2020, May 1). *Revisiting Louisiana's medical legacy: The National Leprosarium in Carville.* Preservation Resource Center of New Orleans. https://prcno.org/revisiting-louisianas-medical-legacy-national-leprosarium-carville/

Georgia woman with flesh-eating disease in "critical" condition. (2012, May 19). Reuters. https://www.reuters.com/article/us-usa-georgia-infection/georgia-woman-with-flesh-eating-disease-in-critical-condition-idUSBRE84I-0EE20120519

Georgiou, A. (2023, March 31). Man loses leg to flesh-eating disease caused by very rare fungus infection. *Newsweek.* https://www.newsweek.com/man-loses-leg-flesh-eating-disease-caused-very-rare-fungus-infection-1791905

Golembiewski, K. (2023, January 25). *What scientists say about the real-life zombie fungi that inspired "The Last of Us."* CNN. https://www.cnn.com/2023/01/25/world/zombie-fungus-ophiocordyceps-the-last-of-us-scn/index.html

Gray, K., Padilla, P., Sparks, B., & Dziewulski, P. (2020). *Distant myonecrosis by atraumatic Clostridium septicum infection in a patient with metastatic breast cancer.* IDCases, 20, e00784. https://doi.org/10.1016/j.idcr.2020.e00784

Guillemin, J. (2006). *Scientists and the history of biological weapons: A brief historical overview of the development of biological weapons in the twentieth century.* EMBO Reports, 7, S45–S49. https://doi.org/10.1038/sj.embor.7400689

Hare, B. (2018, July 23). *Six questions about the brain-eating amoeba, answered.* CNN. https://www.cnn.com/2018/07/23/health/brain-eating-amoeba-hln-somethings-killing-me/index.html

Hassan, S. A., Akhtar, A., Khan, M., Sheikh, F. N., & Asghar, H. (2019). "Frightening" resistant clostridial myonecrosis: A case report. *Cureus,* 11(4). https://doi.org/10.7759/cureus.4539

Held, A. (2017, September 5). *In a case that is "almost impossible," girl dies of malaria in Italy.* NPR. https://www.npr.org/sections/thetwo-way/2017/09/05/548624097/in-a-case-that-is-almost-impossible-girl-dies-of-malaria-in-italy

A history of biological weapons | American experience. PBS. (n.d.). Www.pbs.org. https://www.pbs.org/wgbh/americanexperience/features/weapon-timeline/

The history of leprosy. (n.d.). Leprosy Mission

International. https://www.leprosymission. org/what-is-leprosy/the-history-of-leprosy/

Hoxha, R. (2006). Two Albanians die from black widow spider bites. *BMJ*, 333(7562), 278.2. https://doi.org/10.1136/bmj.333.7562.278-a

Hunt, K. (2023, March 8). *Scientists have revived a "zombie" virus that spent 48,500 years frozen in permafrost.* CNN. https:// www.cnn.com/2023/03/08/world/permafrost-virus-risk-climate-scn/index. html?fbclid=IwAR0ejZoEUpr48bVy_ uh1Wozl6fVKR2laf7e0Yw6EuQsFtTO0w-4YEf7zkTvg

Jankowska, L., Adamski, Z., Polańska, A., Bowszyc-Dmochowska, M., Plagens-Rotman, K., Merks, P., Czarnecka-Operacz, M., & Żaba, R. (2022). Challenges in the diagnosis of tertiary syphilis: Case report with literature review. *International Journal of Environmental Research and Public Health*, 19(24), 16992. https://doi. org/10.3390/ijerph192416992

Jin, L., Fan, K., Liu, S., & Yu, S. (2021). Necrotizing Fasciitis of the jaw, neck and mediastinum caused by Klebsiella oxytoca and Streptococcus constellatus: A case report. *Annals of Palliative Medicine,* 10(7), 8431436–8438436. https:// doi.org/10.21037/apm-20-2427

Kakoullis, L., Pitman, J., Flier, L., & Colgrove, R.

(2022). Fever and ulcerative skin lesions in a patient referred for altered mental status: Clinical and microbiological diagnosis of ulceroglandular tularemia. *Tropical Medicine and Infectious Disease, 7*(9), 220. https://doi.org/10.3390/tropicalmed7090220

A killer toothache?!? Man barely survives traumatic tooth infection. Monsters Inside Me. (2022). In YouTube. https://www.youtube.com/watch?v=dLRShIT1iFs

Kounang, N. (2015, September 14). *How they survived the plague, just barely.* CNN. https://www.cnn.com/2015/09/11/health/plague-survivors/index.html

Lee, B. Y. (2021, October 24). Donovanosis: Why this is called a "flesh eating" sexually transmitted infection. *Forbes.* https://www.forbes.com/sites/brucelee/2021/10/24/donovanosis-why-this-is-called-a-flesh-eating-sexually-transmitted-infection/?sh=77c092f012b4

Leprosy (Hansen's disease): Causes, symptoms & treatment. (2022, May 18). Cleveland Clinic. https://my.clevelandclinic.org/health/diseases/23043-leprosy-hansens-disease

Levs, J., Botelho, G., & Baldwin, B. (2012, May 14). *Family watches "miraculous survival" of woman fighting flesh-eating bacteria.* CNN. https://

www.cnn.com/2012/05/14/health/geor-gia-flesh-eating-bacteria/index.html

Lite, J. (2008, October 8). Medical mystery: Only one person has survived rabies without vaccine--but how? *Scientific American.* https://www.scientificamerican.com/article/jeanna-giese-rabies-survivor/

Lorenzo, M. (2016, January 10). *10 common pathogens that can also eat you away.* Listverse. https://listverse.com/2016/01/10/10-common-patho-gens-that-can-also-eat-you-away/

A man is infected with an African parasitic worm called Loa loa. Monsters Inside Me. Animal Planet. (n.d.). Www.youtube.com. Retrieved April 20, 2023, from https://www.youtube.com/watch?v=IFC2-enWL0g

Maria Bordonado – The freedom to walk again. (n.d.). Www.mediaustralia.com.au. Retrieved April 20, 2023, from https://www.mediaustralia.com.au/patients/patient-stories/elephantiasis/

Marina, S., Broshtilova, V., Botev, I., Guleva, D., Hadzhiivancheva, M., Nikolova, A., & Kazandjieva, J. (2014). Cutaneous mani-festations of toxoplasmosis: A case report. *Serbian Journal of Dermatology and Venereology,* 6(3), 113–119. https://doi.org/10.2478/sjdv-2014-0010

The Manchineel is a scary tropical tree that can kill

you. (2022, September 27). *Southern Living.* https://www.southernliving.com/garden/trees/manchineel-poison-tree

Maurin, M. (2014). Francisella tularensisas a potential agent of bioterrorism? *Expert Review of Anti-Infective Therapy,* 13(2), 141–144. https://doi.org/10.1586/14787210.2015.986463

Maxmen, A. (2015, December 28). *A disease so neglected it's not even on "most-neglected" lists.* NPR. https://www.npr.org/sections/goatsandsoda/2015/12/28/461171017/a-disease-so-neglected-its-not-even-on-most-neglected-lists

Miller, K. (2011, March 8). *Leprosy overview.* WebMD; WebMD. https://www.webmd.com/skin-problems-and-treatments/guide/leprosy-symptoms-treatments-history

Monica's story - Necrotizing Fasciitis. (n.d.). Spauldingrehab.org. Retrieved April 16, 2023, from https://spauldingrehab.org/about/patient-stories/monica

Monsters inside me leprosy - Bing video. (n.d.). Www.bing.com. Retrieved April 14, 2023, from https://www.bing.com/videos/search?q=monsters+inside+me+leprosy&docid=603502841382249427&mid=74811ED4A36552B-D945A74811ED4A36552BD945A&view=detail&FORM=VIRE

Mucormycosis infection: Definition & histopathology.

(2023). Study.com. https://study.com/academy/lesson/mucormycosis-infection-definition-histopathology.html?src=ppc_bing_nonbrand&rcntxt=aws&crt=&kwd=SEO-PPC-ALL&kwid=dat-2329040 505669481:loc-190&agid=12358513025 96746&mt=b&device=c&network=o&_campaign=SeoPPC&msclkid=277210d-7341b155aaac874e720e35133

Mycetoma: A simple thorn prick. (2016, May 22). DNDi. Dndi.org. https://dndi.org/stories/2016/mycetoma-the-faces-of-neglect/

Mycetoma: Hope for a devastating neglected disease. (n.d.). Www.youtube.com. Retrieved April 19, 2023, from https://www.youtube.com/watch?v=kARGZl9s6SQ

The mystery of Anthrax Island and the seeds of death. (2022, February 25). BBC News. https://www.bbc.com/news/uk-scotland-60483849

Newey, S. (2019, September 25). *A glimmer of hope in the fight against a flesh-eating "silent killer."* The Telegraph. https://www.telegraph.co.uk/global-health/science-and-disease/glimmer-hope-fight-against-flesh-eating-silent-killer/

Newman, T. (2018, February 28). *Biological weapons and bioterrorism: Past, present, and future.* Www.medicalnewstoday.com. https://www.medicalnewstoday.com/

articles/321030#Bioterrorism:-Modern-concerns

Nguyen, D. A., Charles, J. E. M., Worrell, J. T., & Wilkes, D. V. (2020). *Cutaneous leishmaniasis in a 65-year-old North Texas male, treated with cryotherapy: A case report.* SAGE Open Medical Case Reports, 8, 2050313X2090459. https://doi.org/10.1177/2050313x20904593

The 1979 anthrax leak | Plague war | FRONTLINE. (n.d.). PBS. Www.pbs.org. https://www.pbs.org/wgbh/pages/frontline/shows/plague/sverdlovsk/#:~:text=On%20April%202%2C%201979%2C%20there

O'Kane, C. (2019, July 13). *Man dies from flesh-eating bacteria 48 hours after Florida beach trip, family says.* Www.cbsnews.com. https://www.cbsnews.com/news/man-dies-from-flesh-eating-bacteria-48-hours-after-florida-beach-trip-family-says-2019-07-13/

Oliver, M. (2014, December 4). *Brown recluse spider bite death of Alabama boy rarer than dying by lightning strike.* Al. https://www.al.com/news/2014/12/brown_recluse_spider_bite_deat.html

Patient story - Living with lymphatic filariasis. (n.d.). Www.youtube.com. Retrieved April 20, 2023, from https://www.youtube.com/watch?v=DPldQtf7_MU

Patient story - understanding lymphatic filariasis. (n.d.). Www.youtube.com. https://www.youtube.com/watch?v=vVZYgkqgOew

Petroni, A. (2021, June 25). *Flesh-eating parasites may be expanding their range as climate heats up.* NPR. https://www.npr.org/sections/health-shots/2021/06/25/1009885640/flesh-eating-parasites-may-be-expanding-their-range-as-climate-heats-up

Pip Stewart on cutaneous leishmaniasis: "It wasn't just the parasite that got under my skin, it was the injustice of it." (2021, October 29). Dndi.org. https://dndi.org/stories/2021/pip-stewart-on-cutaneous-leishmaniasis/

Plane passenger almost lost leg after flesh-eating spider bite. (2015, September 29). The Guardian. https://www.theguardian.com/world/2015/sep/29/barrister-almost-lost-leg-after-flesh-eating-spider-bite

Pneumonia. (2019). https://www.cdc.gov/pneumonia/atypical/psittacosis/index.html

Pruitt, S. (2018, October 4). *When anthrax-laced letters terrorized the nation.* History. https://www.history.com/news/anthrax-attacks-terrorism-letters

Pruitt-Young, S. (2021, November 14). *3 dead, hundreds injured after storms rouse scorpions in Egypt.* NPR. https://www.npr.org/2021/11/14/1055680400/3-dead-hundreds-injured-after-storms-rouse-scorpions-in-egypt

Rabies in humans: Tragic story of Michigan's last death. (2019, October 11). The Detroit News. https://www.detroitnews.com/story/news/local/michigan/2019/10/11/what-happened-last-time-person-died-rabies-michigan/3931347002/

Rinquist, A. (2016, October 27). *10 horrifying tales of flesh-eating diseases.* Listverse. https://listverse.com/2016/10/27/10-horrifying-tales-of-flesh-eating-diseases/

Robinson, O., Sardarizadeh, S., & Horton, J. (2022, March 15). *Ukraine war: Fact-checking Russia's biological weapons claims.* BBC News. https://www.bbc.com/news/60711705

Rodriguez Salamanca, L. (2018, August 19). *Can sick plants make people sick?* Hortnews.extension.iastate.edu. https://hortnews.extension.iastate.edu/2018/10/can-sick-plants-make-people-sick#:~:text=In%20general%2C%20pathogens%20that%20infect

Santhakumar, S. (2022, April 29). *Donovanosis: Definition, causes, symptoms, treatment.* Www.medicalnewstoday.com. https://www.medicalnewstoday.com/articles/flesh-eating-std-donovanosis

Scutti, S., & Christensen, J. (2019, July 1). *A Florida woman dies after surgeries to cure her flesh-eating bacteria infection.* CNN. https://www.cnn. com/2019/07/01/health/flesh-eating-flori- da-woman-trnd/index.html

Shakhnazarova, N. (2019, December 10). *Terrifying new species of spider can rot human flesh with single bite and hides in furniture.* The US Sun. https://www.the-sun.com/news/142851/ terrifying-new-species-of-spider-can-rot-hu- man-flesh-with-single-bite-and-hides-in-furni- ture/#:~:text=Loxosceles%20Tenochtitlan%20 spiders%3F-

Sharma, S. (2022, November 3). *Boy dies from multi- ple cardiac arrests after scorpion sting while put- ting on shoe.* The Independent. https://www. independent.co.uk/news/world/americas/bra- zil-boy-heart-attack-scorpion-sting-b2215740. html

Sita's story - Visceral leishmaniasis in India - Reaching a billion. (n.d.). Uniting to Combat NTDs. Retrieved April 18, 2023, from https://uni- tingtocombatntds.org/reports/5th-report/ sita-story/

Strickland, N. H. (2000). My most unfortunate ex- perience: Eating a manchineel "beach ap- ple." *BMJ, 321*(7258), 428–428. https://doi. org/10.1136/bmj.321.7258.428

Sukel, K. (2007, May 21). *Cerebral malaria, a wily foe.*

Dana Foundation. https://dana.org/article/
cerebral-malaria-a-wily-foe/

*Symptoms, transmission, and current treatments for cu-
taneous leishmaniasis.* (2020, March 17).
DNDi. Dndi.org. https://dndi.org/diseases/
cutaneous-leishmaniasis/facts/

Thomas, L. (2017, January 26). *History of leprosy.*
News-Medical.net. https://www.news-medical.
net/health/History-of-leprosy.aspx

Tobin, E. H., & Jih, W. W. (2001). Sporotrichoid lym-
phocutaneous infections: Etiology, diagnosis
and therapy. *American Family Physician,* 63(2),
326–333. https://www.aafp.org/pubs/afp/is-
sues/2001/0115/p326.html

Tucson family has personal ties to new scorpion treatment.
(2011, August 4). Https://Www.kold.com.
https://www.kold.com/story/15206343/new-
treatment-for-scorpion-stings-has-personal-
ties-for-one-family/

Vollmer, M. E., & Glaser, C. (2016). A Balamuthia
survivor. *JMM Case Reports,* 3(3). https://doi.
org/10.1099/jmmcr.0.005031

What is rabies? (2019). Centers for Disease Control and
Prevention. https://www.cdc.gov/rabies/about.
html

Xu, L.-Q., Zhao, X.-X., Wang, P.-X., Yang, J., & Yang,
Y.-M. (2019). Multidisciplinary treatment of
a patient with Necrotizing Fasciitis caused by

Staphylococcus aureus: A case report. *World Journal of Clinical Cases*, 7(21), 3595–3602. https://doi.org/10.12998/wjcc.v7.i21.3595

Yeap, W. (2019). Fatal neck Necrotizing Fasciitis caused by hypermucoviscous Klebsiella pneumoniae. *Crit Care Shock,* 22(1). https://criticalcareshock. org/files/2019/01/fatal-neck-necrotizing-fas- ciitis-caused-by-hypermucoviscous-klebsiel- la-pneumoniae.pdf

Young girl survives bubonic plague—Monsters Inside Me. (2023). In YouTube. https://www.youtube. com/watch?v=xPgzlO0SIQs

Zeaiter, N., Maassarani, D., Ghanime, G., & Sleiman, Z. (2022). A case report of rapidly Necrotizing Fasciitis post-falling down treated reconstruc- tively. *Cureus*, 14(8). https://doi.org/10.7759/ cureus.28055

About the Author

J.D. Sherwood is a clinical laboratory scientist with over 30 years of experience in the field. She holds a master's degree in quality assurance and is passionate about learning and growing through reading and education. In addition to her professional pursuits, J.D. enjoys world travel and cherishes her relationships with her daughter and her wonderful boyfriend. She believes in living life to the fullest and making the most of every day.

Printed in Great Britain
by Amazon